THE ILLUSION OF LOVE

T0373065

The Illusion of Love

*Why the
Battered Woman
Returns to
Her Abuser*

David P. Celani

Columbia University Press · *New York*

Columbia University Press
New York   Chichester, West Sussex
Copyright © 1994 Columbia University Press

Library of Congress Cataloging-in-Publication Data

Celani, David P.
   The illusion of love : why the battered woman returns to her
abuser / David P. Celani.
       p.   cm.
   Includes bibliographical references and index.

   ISBN 978-0-231-10036-6 (cloth)   ISBN 978-0-231-10037-3 (paper)

   1. Abused women—Psychology.   2. Object relations (Psychoanalysis)
3. Codependency.   I. Title.
RC569.5.F3C45 1994
616.85'822—dc20   94-29717
                                                                                        CIP

Casebound editions of Columbia University Press books are printed on
permanent and durable acid-free paper.

Printed in the United States of America

to Veronica

and

to the memory of my mother

It is hardly possible to exaggerate the lovelessness in which most people live, men or women: wanting love, unable to give it, or inspire it, unable to keep it if they get it, not knowing how to treat it, lacking the humility, or the very love itself that could teach them how to love: it is the painfullest thing in human life, and, since love is purely a creation of the human imagination, it is merely perhaps the most important of all examples of how the imagination continually outruns the creature it inhabits . . . Having imagined love, we are condemned to its perpetual disappointment; or so it seems.

Katherine Anne Porter, *Orpheus in Purgatory*

CONTENTS

My introduction to the world of self-destructive human relationships came during the first years of my practice. Day after day I listened to one patient after another describe the humiliation, rejection, and criticism that they were subjected to by family members whom they loved. It was painfully obvious to me that the majority of my patients' problems were based on their need for, and loyalty to, members of their immediate families, who rejected them time after time. Other patients suffered from a similar problem, but at a different stage of life: they were attached to adult partners, most often husbands or wives, who constantly demeaned, exploited, and criticized them. I simply could not understand why my apparently normal patients did not leave these negative and self-destructive relationships. When I finally bluntly asked why they refused to give up on family members or adult partners, and suggested that they develop new relationships outside the current destructive situation, the response was most often outrage and incredulity. I was lectured that "blood was thicker than water" and that "family" meant "forever," regardless of how badly any particular individual was being treated. Clearly I had hit an extremely sensitive nerve. My patients' dependence on their families was so extreme that the destructive attachment had to be rationalized and defended with almost religious fervor. This indicated that they could not lose the relationship without going into a state of psychological collapse, despite the fact that many of their families behaved in the most profoundly vicious and undermining ways.

Several years later, I began the challenging work of treating battered women along with my other patients. I had already learned that many of my female patients had been physically abused at some time in their lives. I found that battered women had very similar histories to, and were no different psychologically from, my other patients in their attraction to and dependence upon partners who rejected them—*except* that they were being physically beaten. Once again, I had difficulty understanding why these seemingly normal women would go back to men who violently beat them.

Much to my surprise, my desperate and needy battered female patients were suspicious and mistrustful of my heartfelt attempts to aid them. Conversely, they were completely gullible and easily duped by their abusers. These patients seemed to have a fine-tuned interpersonal radar that would detect and seek out the one potential abuser in a roomful of healthy men. Again, I was unprepared for what I was observing; I had no explanation for it, since my training in academic psychology almost completely ignored the topic of unconscious attachment to abusive partners. By contrast, popular psychology seemed to have one new answer after another for physically and emotionally abused women who were unable to leave their adult partners. These relationships were described endlessly in self-help books, with a whole host of recently coined terms (none of which was explanatory), including "co-dependency," "enmeshment," "love-addiction," and the "trauma bond."

The key event in my career came in 1983, when I discovered the work of W. R. D. Fairbairn, a Scottish analyst who wrote about the effects of neglect and unmet dependency needs on the personality development of children. I was astonished to discover that his papers on personality structure and development, which were published between 1940 and 1960, exactly explained why my patients returned again and again to those who demeaned and abused them. The accuracy and power of Fairbairn's model came directly from his experience working in a public orphanage, where he saw the explosive results when children were forcibly separated from their parents. Such separation wasn't considered an important psychological event in the 1940s, when psychiatry was dominated by the Freudian model of human development. Fairbairn's great gift was that he did not allow his training as a Freudian analyst to obscure what he saw. His model was carefully constructed around his observation that abused, neglected, and abandoned children were, paradoxically, more attached to their parents than were normal children. This psychological model saw early events in the relationship between the infant and its caregiver as the fundamental building blocks of the developing child's personality. Fairbairn's model of personality development details the inner mechanisms responsible for the child's attachment and loyalty to parents who have, in reality, abused and neglected him. This book applies Fairbairn's basic principles to the adult equivalent of childhood dependence on rejecting parents, which in its most extreme form is the battered woman's dependence on her abuser. Thus, I extend modern psychoanalytic theory to the scenario of domestic abuse.

Three years have passed since I began writing *The Illusion of Love*, and during that short period there has been an explosion of interest in Fairbairn's writings. In October 1996 the first conference in the United States devoted entirely to the work of this psychoanalytic pioneer will take place. At least ten new books on Fairbairn's work, including a two-volume compendium of all his writings, have been published in the past three years. What has happened to suddenly make a theory of personality first introduced in 1940 so popular? The answer, in a word, is that Fairbairn's model of personality development has proven to be more consistently accurate than the prevailing Freudian model. This reality took a relatively long time to be accepted because of resistance from many psychoanalytically trained psychologists and psychiatrists who have remained loyal to Freud's ideas. Many simply refused to consider Fairbairn's work, as it represented a huge threat to the Freudian model. The two models are mutually exclusive: that is, either Freud or Fairbairn is right, but not both. I describe the basic differences between the models in chapter 1.

Thus, part of this book describes a contest between different explanatory models, each of which claims to illuminate the dynamics and mechanisms that lead women to remain in life-endangering relationships. This contest is enormously important. Competing theories organize our perceptions of events differently, and the most widely accepted model becomes the basis for treatment, efforts at prevention, and ultimately for social policy.

I have made the human ego the focus of this book, and each chapter looks at a different aspect of this powerful psychological construct. The ego is a concept used to describe the aspect of the human personality that contains our view and opinions of ourselves and of the people around us. The ego also contains a set of emotional and cognitive skills that, under the proper developmental conditions, matures to produce what we collectively consider to be a fully functioning adult personality. Chapter 2 focuses on the human ego during childhood and describes various parental behaviors that can severely inhibit the development of mature ego functions. Chapter 3 describes, in terms of overt behavior, the effects of malformed and immature ego structures. Those individuals with insufficient ego structures are diagnostically described as having character or personality disorders. Chapter 4 focuses on two of Fairbairn's key contributions to the field, the concepts of the moral defense and the splitting defense, the two major defense mechanisms that children and adults use to remain attached to their frustrating parents or partners. Chapter 5 applies all the material in the previous chapters to the analysis of Lenore Walker's "cycle theory of violence." This theory is a description of the three typical stages of the battering cycle, and I apply Fairbairn's principles to explain the unconscious dynamics behind each of the three stages. Finally, in chapter 6, I outline a treatment program for the battered woman, using a model designed to strengthen the ego structure of the victim of abuse.

This model focuses on involuntary, unconscious participation by the female victim of abuse and has not been applied to the battering scenario up until now. The analysis of the ego structures of both participants in the battering scenario offers a more complex understanding of the basis of physical abuse than does the popular current theory. This analysis also describes the types of psychological mechanisms and defenses, developed only in childhood, that are the typical antecedents to victimization in adulthood. The sad reality is that battering (as defined by two or more incidents of physical abuse) happens only to women who have been seriously deprived in childhood. The adult woman who is the repeated victim of physical abuse has been *twice* deprived, because her childhood experiences did not allow the development of a healthy ego structure, and this forces her to compromise in her choice of men.

For those readers looking for blame, there is plenty to go around, but it is not directed at the victims of abuse (and paradoxically, not at the perpetrators either) but at a culture that values children so little (and parental rights so much) that we blindly allow child abuse and deprivation to continue. We are then outraged and surprised when our erstwhile child-victim becomes either an abuser or a victim of abuse in adulthood. My goal is to present the reader with a more accurate model of the battering scenario, in the hope of stimulating better forms of treatment and more enlightened social policy that focus on the prevention of this most preventable of human tragedies.

ACKNOWLEDGMENTS

The writing of this book was supported by many friends and colleagues. First, I extend warmest thanks to Henry Grinberg, Ph.D., who used both his training in psychoanalysis and his expertise as an editor to critique much of the manuscript. I also extend thanks to George W. Albee, Ph.D., who has supported my work over many years, and who spent hours reading the many versions of the manuscript. I am also again indebted to Robert Barasch, Ph.D., who applied his skills, both theoretical and editorial, to much of the manuscript. I am also grateful to Gioia Stevens, of Columbia University Press, who was patient and enthusiastic throughout the project. And finally, I again express my appreciation to my wife, Veronica, who has comforted and sustained me during this project and many others.

The Illusion of Love

INTRODUCTION

America is awash in an epidemic of violence toward women. It has probably always been so; however, until recently it's been a poorly kept secret. The June 17, 1992, issue of the *Journal of the American Medical Association* sounded a call to all American physicians to alert themselves to the crisis of physical spousal abuse that pours into the emergency rooms of this country on a daily basis. The summary of the lead article from this journal began with the following statement:

> Evidence collected over the last 20 years indicates that physical and sexual violence against women is an enormous problem. Much of this violence is perpetrated by women's intimate partners or in relationships that would presumably carry some protective aura (e.g., father-daughter, boyfriend-girlfriend). This violence carries with it both short- and long-term sequelae for women and affects both their physical and psychological well-being.
>
> (Browne 1992:3184)

The article goes on to describe the astounding number of women affected by physical and sexual violence. Spousal violence is not an isolated phenomenon, nor is it limited to the lower socioeconomic classes. The violence that these women experience is not mild, but rather brutal and recurrent:

Studies now document that women in the United States are more likely to be assaulted and injured, raped, or killed by a current or ex-male partner than by all other types of assailants combined. In a 1985 survey of intact couples, nearly one out of every eight husbands has carried out one or more acts of physical aggression against their female partner during the survey year. Over one third of these assaults involved severe aggression such as punching, kicking, choking, beating up, or using a knife or a gun. In an average 12-month period in the United States, approximately 2 million women are severely assaulted by male partners . . . Further, victims of violence by intimates are much more likely to be reassaulted within 6 months than are those attacked by nonintimates.

(Browne 1992:3185)

There are two major questions embedded within these statements that call out for answers. The first is why do so many men perpetrate assaults on the women whom they supposedly love? The second, perhaps more compelling, is why do women who are beaten return, often again and again, to the very same abusive relationship? This book is an attempt to answer these two fundamental questions.

The answers to these two questions are not apparent to many of us in this society, including the very physicians who treat the injuries of abused women. One of the primary findings reported in a separate study in the same issue of the *Journal of the American Medical Association* was that physicians who were confronted with patients that were badly beaten by their spouses or partners treated only the physical injuries of the patient but avoided open discussion of the source of the injuries. Their reasons for this avoidance was summed up in the phrase "Pandora's box."

Repeatedly, the image of opening Pandora's box was used by physicians to describe their reactions to exploring domestic violence with their patients. This metaphor suggests the fear of unleashing a myriad of evils. By examining the comments of the respondents, these "evils" began to take the shape of "too close for comfort," "fear of offending," "powerlessness," "loss of control," and the "tyranny of time" (Sugg and Inui 1992).

The authors go on to explain that many physicians were closely identified with their patients and had difficulty believing that persons from the same socioeconomic class were at risk for domestic violence. In addition, more than 50 percent of the physicians in this same study reported that they were inhibited about discussing family violence for fear of offending the patient by prying into a matter that they saw as "private." Other factors that inhibited the physicians were their sense of powerlessness to do anything about the situation in which these women were immersed and their perception that the outcome of their interventions was in the hands of the patient. That is, unlike most medical procedures, where the patient's motivation is irrelevant (such as when intervening with penicillin), the escape from domestic violence required active participation by the patient. Finally, these physicians also recognized that effective intervention would require far more than the normal twenty-minute examination.

If physicians are avoidant of and unprepared to deal with family violence, then what can we expect from individual members of the general public? Like the physicians, we all have trouble believing persons like ourselves could be the victims of domestic violence. Like the physicians, we are exceedingly fearful of prying into others' private lives, and we have a sense of powerlessness when confronted by the specter of domestic violence. It is a terribly complex problem involving many individuals, and very few of us have the tools to tackle it head on. We are all wary of situations where we can only help others indirectly. We tend to avoid involvement in situations that have the potential to go on and on, swamping the help giver with continuing, insatiable demands. Intervention into this complex, frightening, often hard-to-believe world of domestic violence is enormously time-consuming, and there is no guarantee that the effort will result in success.

Hopefully this book will serve physicians, mental health providers, and others who are interested in the underlying psychology of abuse by providing basic guidelines written in terms that professionals and laypeople alike can understand. My goal is to reduce the mystery, fear, and misinformation that surround the phenomenon of domestic violence.

The Paradox of the Return to the Rejecting Partner

The most puzzling aspect of the battering scenario is the often observed return of the victim to the batterer after a severe beating. The mystery of this apparently irrational behavior is reduced if it is understood as standing on the extreme end of a continuum of a large variety of behaviors, all of which involve the return of one person to others who are (more or less) abusive or rejecting. For example, the milder forms of this pattern of returning to those that disappoint us are described almost endlessly in the self-help literature, in such popular books as Robin Norwood's *Women Who Love Too Much*, Susan Forward's *Men That Hate Women and the Women That Love Them*, and Cowan and Kinder's *Smart Women, Foolish Choices*. This variation of the return to the rejecting person occurs under the cover of romance and love, and these books focus on women who return to rejecting men.

A second, related form of the return to the rejecting "other" occurs with both genders in (now) adult children who were neglected and abused during their childhoods. Contrary to logic these "adults" often end up either living with or constantly visiting their parents while neglecting or avoiding other more appropriate adult relationships. Almost unbelievably, these adults (often my patients) return, again and again, to the very parents who failed them in the first place. These adult children go back to parents who used to be physically abusive, parents who now endlessly criticize and disparage them. Naturally not every adult child of abusive parents has living parents to return to. Many of my patients with deceased parents manage to find new individuals, spouses, friends, or relatives who treat them as badly as did their original parents. My experience as a psychologist has convinced me that the greatest challenge to persons with unsatisfactory and dysfunctional backgrounds is to escape from the very people who frustrated them in childhood, or in other cases to avoid new individuals with the same negative and destructive characteristics as their original frustrating and depriving parents. The pattern of returning again and again to a rejecting parent or partner is the prototype of the return to a partner who is physically abusive. These behaviors are psychologically identical, and differ only in degree of severity.

The endless struggle with rejections from childhood, and the ensuing compulsion of the rejected child-adult to return to the persons who rejected them is a topic that is not limited to the field of psychology. Novelists have also used the child's attachment to abusive parents as a major theme, as in the case of Philip Roth's novel *Portnoy's Complaint*. This novel is centered on the endless agony experienced by the protagonist, Alexander Portnoy, over the rejections that he experienced from his manipulative mother. When we

look at this novel closely we will see that Portnoy cannot free himself from his mother's influence over his life because she is so deeply
embedded in his psyche.

A Theory of the Victim's Return to the Abuser

Academic theory, specifically psychoanalytic theory, does have one
writer who championed the attachment of the rejected individual to
the rejecter as the core issue of mental health, a Scottish psychoanalyst named W. R. D. Fairbairn. He worked in what would now be
called a public orphanage from 1927 to 1935, and noticed that children who were forcibly removed from their abusive homes remained
extraordinarily attached, both in fantasy and in reality, to their parents. This is a difficult observation to accept, for one would expect
just the opposite result. That is, one would expect that children that
were beaten or abused would be fearful, avoidant, and eager to escape
from their parents. Fairbairn became interested in this extraordinary
attachment, and he questioned the children about the abuses that
had occurred in their homes. He was astonished to discover that
these abused children insisted that their parents were good, and that
they themselves were the cause of all the family problems. These
two observations led Fairbairn to construct a psychological model in
which emotional disorder was seen as based on the attachment of
children to their abusing or neglectful parents.

It is a rather long trip from Fairbairn's orphanage to the battered
woman of today; however that is the territory that will be covered in
this book. The discoveries and observations produced by this one
obscure but brilliant analyst will yield the reasons that otherwise
"sane" adults (both women and men) remain in, and return to, abusing relationships (both emotionally frustrating and physically abusive)
even though they are exposed to rejection and violence again and
again. There is a tangible air of emergency around the issue of spouse
abuse, and the reader may wish for the Explanation on the very first
page. In reality the psychological processes underlying the uniquely
human attachment to those who abuse and demean us are complex,
and there are competing theories that claim to have the most convincing analysis. It is important for the reader to understand the dif-

ferent theories, and to examine the interpretations they offer for the battering behavior that exists in the relationships of men and women.

I want to begin this journey of explanation by presenting a typical case example of a patient who returned again and again to rejecting "others." The gender of the patient is male, and I chose a male patient to illustrate the very real fact that the return to the rejecting "other" occurs in males as well as in females, and moreover, that these milder forms of the return to rejecting partners are related to the return of the battered victim to her abuser. When we fully understand why John went back repeatedly to women who exploited him, we will have a viable explanation for more serious variations on the same theme: the return of the battering victim to her abuser.

John was a forty-year-old cabinet and furniture maker who came to me in deep distress. His early childhood in rural New England was sad and extremely lonely. His father was a college professor who spent the majority of his nonworking hours locked in his den listening to opera. His mother was an intensely frustrated and demanding woman who used John as the "man" of the household since her husband was unavailable to her. The relationship between John and his mother was far from pleasant, as he could never seem to do enough for her. As an adult he never married, but rather had a series of "relationships" with demanding women. During our first therapy session he described the endless troubles he was having with his partner, Sue, in whose house he lived. John complained incessantly that Sue was selfish, self-centered, and unreasonable, but somehow he could not bring himself to leave her. She ran a horse boarding and training business that was very successful. She had two children by a prior marriage, Toby, fourteen, and Jean, seventeen, who both actively participated in the running of the stable. Sue was on the road nearly every weekend, showing her customers horses at various events. Jean was in charge of the daily exercise and training schedule, while Toby did barn cleaning and feeding of the dozen horses they boarded. John's role was to tow horses nearly every weekend to the various competitions, groom the horses that were being shown, order all the supplies, and feed and supervise the extra help. The only flaw in this cooperative scenario was that John hated and feared horses, and had a full-time job designing and building custom furniture. It appeared to him that his needs were being swept away by his partner's needs, which were dominating his whole life. Despite his unhappiness with the situation, he put up with it, paid half the rent, cooked for everyone, and allowed his woodworking business to slowly fall by the wayside. John came to therapy because this was the third time this type of situation had arisen in his life. He had finally become so distressed by the frustration he was experiencing that he was willing to risk looking at this repeated pattern with an outside observer.

John had met Sue through his prior girlfriend, Gail, a successful interior decorator, who had redecorated Sue's home. At that time John was helping Gail with her business and had come to Sue's house to install curtains. John had been living with Gail and her daughter for three years, but he was becoming increasingly upset by Gail's emotional outbursts and threats to break up their relationship. Despite this he had put his career in furniture making on hold in order to help Gail out. As time went on he felt that his needs had become secondary to Gail's increasing demands, which had taken over as the guiding force in his life. He was also acting as the father to Gail's daughter Christine, who needed special attention because of a learning disability. In fact, he was spending far more time with Chris and her educational needs than Gail was. The opportunity arose during the redecoration job to engage in a heated affair with Sue, which was another repeated trend in John's life. Within two months he moved out of Gail's house and into Sue's, without ever living on his own. At forty-years-old he was saddled with debt, owned no property, and had a career that never seemed to get off the ground.

John's work with me eventually gave him enough strength to move out "on his own" for the first extended period of his life. This occurred after several years of work in therapy, during which he gained emotional distance from Sue. John discovered, to his surprise, that he really disliked his ex-girlfriend Sue "as a person," because of her selfish use of her children, himself, and nearly anyone else with whom she came into contact. It distressed him to recognize he had become so completely dependent on Sue that he had to hide from the reality that he disliked her. Soon after moving out on his own his prior girlfriend, Gail, reentered his life, and he came dangerously close to moving back with her, thus indicating that he was not yet ready to be out "on his own."

We will begin our explanation of John's return to women who exploited him with a brief introduction to psychological models or theories that purport to explain the repeated pattern seen in persons who return to people who frustrate them endlessly.

CHAPTER ONE

Three Psychological Models of Human Functioning

The field of personality development is fragmented into many warring theoretical camps because there is no absolute agreement as to how humans function psychologically. There is disagreement about what motivates humankind, as well as the factors that are most important in human development. Some theorists speculate that the development of language is the key to understanding the development of the child, others believe the development of logic is crucial, learning theorists point to complex sequences of learned responses, classical Freudians believe that biologically based drives are the basic motivators, and so on. When we are faced with a lack of empirical knowledge, theories come into play, since they are the next best thing to absolute knowledge.

Let us look at the ability to predict the weather as an introduction to the role of scientific models. In prescientific times the weather was assumed to be controlled by spirits. This primitive model is not completely out of style, for here in my state of Vermont the thickness of the coat of certain woolly caterpillars is often used as an indicator of future weather patterns. The major competing model for weather prediction is based on the scientific observations of temperature, humidity, and barometric pressure. These observations are combined with the *model*, which is knowledge of the dynamics of weather-related phenomena—i.e., that low pressure systems rotate counter-clockwise, that highs circulate clockwise, and that the jet stream moves from west to east. Just a few observations and a small knowledge of nature's dynamics put the meteorologist way ahead of the proponents of the woolly caterpillar model when it comes to understanding and predicting what type of weather the next day will bring. The two models are poorly matched. However the point I would like to make is that some models do a much better job of understanding the observations, and therefore of predicting the future, than do others. I will review the most important psychological models that have contributed to our understanding of what Fairbairn called the "return to the bad object," and the reader will be able to tell for him or herself which model fits the data that we know as domestic abuse. Once again, we must use theories to explain domestic abuse because no one has absolute knowledge as to why this tragic pattern emerges in human relationships.

Sigmund Freud and the "Psychodynamic Model"

Let us quickly review the first and most influential psychological model of human functioning that we have known to date: Freud's model of psychodynamics. I am starting with Freud because Fairbairn's work emerged from Freud's prior discoveries about human neurosis, and Fairbairn developed his model as an extension of Freud's original work. Furthermore, many of Freud's original concepts are used by most of us in the mental health field, including the concept of the unconscious, the ego defenses such as repression, and the overall focus on the individual's childhood as the key to his or her adult problems. Finally, one of the current explanations of the return of the abused woman to her abuser comes from a peripheral part of Freud's original model, called repetition compulsion, and this concept will be examined in chapter 4.

Freud chose sexuality as the key motivational factor in human development. Many now think that this was an error, but Freud was very clever and deliberate in his choice. He wrote during the period from 1895 to his death in 1939. The most famous scientist of Freud's era was Charles Darwin, whose theory of evolution produced a (nonpsychological) model of man that challenged the most potent and widespread explanation for the existence of humankind on earth—the religious/creationist model. Darwin's theory of the appearance of human life on earth assumed that we had evolved from, and were related to, other and earlier forms of life. Darwin's science-based challenge to the creationist model increased the status of scientific thought enormously. He demonstrated that scientific thought could become the most influential category of thought of that time.

Freud was vastly influenced by Darwin's discoveries, which emphasized modern man's debt to his ancient past. Freud was very interested in ancient cultures, evidenced by the fact that he was both an avid collector of antiquities and a reader of mythology. He desperately wanted to be known and accepted as a scientist of the status that Darwin had attained. His ambition, his natural inclination toward ancient peoples, and his belief that biology was the most important of all sciences played major roles in his model. Freud, although a medical doctor, had devoted much of his early career to research on muscle and nerve tissue, and had made a name for himself by discovering new and better techniques of dyeing cells for study. Biology was central to his life, and amazingly he did not begin the line of thought that evolved into the model that he called psychoanalysis until he was almost forty years old.

It is not surprising that Freud's model of human psychological functioning is based on biology and closely allied with Darwin. He centered his model on the concept of the *id*, which linked the psychic structure of "modern" humans back to primitive forebears. The id is Freud's translation of Darwin's theory of evolution into a psychological concept. Freud theorized that each human had inside him/her a biological storehouse of primitive drives that had been present in earlier human forms. He assumed that the id was comprised of all instinctualized drives and primitive sexualized energy, which he called *libidinal energy*, or *libido*. The id was assumed to seek out pleasure and avoid tension. Thus it operated on the *pleasure principle*, seeking to find pathways to discharge sexually based impulses. Because it is unconscious, the id was assumed to have no regard for, or contact with, reality. Freud's model of psychological development focused on the gradual maturation and transformation of this primitive sexualized energy as it moved through the child's body during four interestingly named hypothetical developmental stages (oral, anal, phallic, and genital). These transformations change id energy into a more complex form called the *ego*, or *ego structure*. The ego in Freud's model is a servant that is charged with getting the id's biological needs (called "drives" by Freud) met in socially acceptable ways. The ego was conceptualized by Freud as a mechanism that had good contact with reality and operated on the *reality principle*. The ego has access to both the desires of the id as well as the constraints of society. Thus, the ego's role is that of a middleman that assesses the internal demands of the id and then makes "deals" with the world to get those unconscious needs met.

The final internal component in Freud's model is called the *superego*, and it is the last to emerge. This component is comprised of remembered parental and societal teaching regarding morality and altruism, and, like the ego, it too is well organized. As one can imagine, this component is often in conflict with the id, and it pressures the ego to conform to its demands. Thus the ego is impinged upon by both sides, and its role is to accommodate these warring intrapsychic components. The eternal struggle between these opposed components is the source of the word "dynamic," which describes the ever changing inner landscape.

Let me use a simple example. A young man stops his car at a stoplight. Deep in his unconscious, the aggressive id energy demands, "Drive through it, don't stop for anything." However, this command from the basement of the psyche is screened by the ego, which is mostly concerned about the reality issues at stake. The ego may take the id's demand into consideration, but it is inhibited by the fear of getting a traffic ticket. The superego is also pressuring the ego from upstairs, pointing out how it is immoral and bad for society if all drivers were to disobey the rules. Thus our hapless ego is pressured from both sides, and it must be robust if it is to fight off primitive impulses from the id or excessively moralistic injunctions from the superego.

For Freud the basic developmental conflict lies between the primitive biological forces within the id and the constraints of the newly crowded industrialized world in which "modern man" found himself. When early humans lived in the outdoors surrounded by physical dangers, it is possible that the primitive id acted as a biological advantage in maintaining high rates of reproduction and therefore of survival. For instance, aggression and a powerful sexual drive in both men and women might insure a certain amount of safety from predators and a large number of offspring. Aggression in women also might have served to protect the children from misdirected violence from the male toward them. Conversely, ego-mediated behaviors, such as good table manners or appropriate toileting habits, were of little value to primitive survival-based cultures. This model contains no mention of the effects of human attachment on the development of personality or on the establishment of society, a critical omission that has led to the many modifications of classical Freudian theory.

I have used the concept *ego structure* a number of times without defining it for the reader. What is a "structure" and what does "structural" change mean? A structure in Freud's model is one of the three components of the psyche, the id, the ego, and, later, the superego. To make things more confusing, these three components are more or less organized—or, "structured." Thus the word *structured* means compartmentalized, organized, containing plans, pathways, functions, or strategies. To reduce the confusion I will substitute the word *component* to denote the three parts of the psyche, and the word *structured* will be used only to indicate the relative complexity of the separate components. For instance, the id is a component assumed to be primitive (poorly organized) and structureless in that it contains no plans, strategies, or categories of experience; rather, it is a pool of energy seeking expression in either aggression or sexuality. The ego is a component that is (after full development) just the opposite, in that it has a series of functions, concepts, plans, and strategies all designed to meet the needs of the id.

Psychological Trauma and the Mystery of "Railroad Spine"

Psychological disorders were studied by many physicians before Freud came on the scene. The early models of psychological dysfunction assumed that nervous disorders originated with events that overwhelmed the individual's capacity to cope with the trauma. Drinka (1984) described a number of pre-Freudian explanations of neurosis, many of which came from examination of people who had been traumatized by train accidents. Freud's time saw the expansion of the railroad system in Europe as part of industrial revolution. Trains were feared by the rural peasants, who were in transition to new lives as workers in cities. Railroad travel was both unreliable and dangerous, as the technology was new and derailments were commonplace. Soon the railroads were being sued by large numbers of injured patrons with both physical and psychological injuries. The railroads then hired physicians to examine injured claimants to assess the extent of the physical injuries and to differentiate those with "hysterias" from those with actual physical injuries. In the 1880s many vague and diverse disorders that originated from traumas due to railroad accidents were nicknamed "railroad spine," for it was assumed that the spinal cord had somehow been injured, while later they were considered to be hysterias. At that time *hysteria* was a general term that was used to describe fainting spells, excessive fears, delirium, unexplained weakness, and nervous exhaustion.

Two of these railroad physicians were Herbert Page, who worked for the London and Northwest Railway in Great Britain, and Hermann Oppenheim of Berlin. Page wrote a book in 1883 on injuries to the spine, and in it he described two hundred cases that appeared to be psychologically based hysterias. Oppenheim did not believe that there was any injury to the spine and instead coined the term *traumatic neurosis*, a concept that is now associated with Freud but existed prior to his theory. There was wide debate on the cause of neurosis, but all the early models involved the concept of psychological trauma that was assumed to have overpowered the delicate nervous systems of the sufferers.

Freud was influenced by the existing models of his era, and he joined the trauma bandwagon by incorporating psychological shock as a significant part of his model. One of his earliest cases, described in his first book, *Studies on Hysteria* (1895), which he coauthored with Joseph Breuer, was the case of Katharina, an eighteen-year-old waitress who served him in an inn while he was on a hiking vacation. She described a sudden shortness of breath, buzzing sensations, and feeling a heavy weight pressing on her chest. Freud noted that he could not get away from neuroses, even when hiking at six thousand feet, and he examined the young woman. Freud immediately guessed that sexuality had played a key role in the symptoms: "I had found often enough that in girls anxiety was a consequence of the horror by which a virginal mind is overcome when it is faced for the first time with the world of sexuality" (127). In fact, this was the case with Katharina, who reported that she had looked through a window and seen her uncle in a sexual embrace with a young female employee of the inn. This vision overwhelmed her and made her feel dizzy and out of breath. She then became sick to her stomach for three days, which Freud interpreted as a physical expression of her disgust at the scene she had viewed. Freud also uncovered the fact that this same uncle had made sexual approaches to Katharina when she was fourteen. Freud analyzed her symptom of shortness of breath as a pared down version of her earlier vomiting. Here we have classic example of early neurosis:

1. a sexually based conflict between the id, which was assumed to be aroused by the sexual scene, and the superego, which was assumed to demand that it be repressed,
2. a sudden trauma that overwhelmed a delicate constitution and,
3. a clear and obvious symptom that was linked symbolically to the incident.

Freud's model fit the problems of his time.

Times have changed since the case of Katharina, but do such traumatic neuroses occur today? In fact, they do occasionally crop up, as the following example of Annie Perry illustrates:

On Easter eve, 1944, Edward Leon Cameron, a prosperous 34-year-old farmer, disappeared from his home in Raeford, N.C. . . . Now, Cameron's oldest daughter, Mrs. Annie Blue Perry, who was 9 years old at the time, has agonizingly discovered what happened to her father 35 years ago. The bizarre mystery began to unravel more than a year ago when Perry, now 45, an associate professor of reading skills at Valencia Community College in Orlando, Fla., sought psychiatric help for her continuing emotional problems. Probing her childhood during therapy, she mentioned a haunting memory of her missing father's bloodstained body. Encouraged by her psychiatrist, she contacted the FBI with her story. She then returned to North Carolina to help with the investigation and even met twice with a local hypnotist, state Sen. Joseph Raynor. In her trances, she recounted even more grisly sights to local authorities. Her parents had quarreled that night, Perry remembered. The next morning, she saw her mother in the kitchen and the sink full of bloody pots and pans. "I asked her what had happened, and she said she'd hurt herself, but there was too much blood," Perry told Raynor. . . . During the day, Perry recalled, she saw her mother go repeatedly into a rarely used front bedroom. While her mother was out, Perry looked in and saw her father's body on the floor—naked, except for bloodsoaked gauze around his groin. "He's not breathing. I think he's dead," she said in her trance. . . . A few days later,

when she went to the family outhouse, she saw her father's face
partially submerged in the pool of excrement.

(Beck and Caroll 1979:37)

This example illustrates a modern-day traumatic neurosis in which
the psyche of the child became overwhelmed by the experiences that
she encountered. Her solution to this trauma was to repress these
memories. Over time these memories pushed upward into her
awareness in the form of her symptoms, which were remnants of the
memories of seeing her father's body. The only element in this case
that is at variance with Freud's early formulations is the sexuality
issue. There was nothing sexual in her memories, however, instead
there appears a second, more potent human motivator: Annie's
dependency on her mother. She *had to* repress the murder scene
because if she had remembered it, this memory would have placed
her in grave danger of losing her one remaining parent. That is, if
Annie had told a teacher or friend what she had seen, her mother
would have been jailed, and Annie would have lost both parents at
nine years of age. Repression saved her from this abandonment and
kept her mother with her. One could hypothesize that the memories
emerged only when Annie could psychologically afford to live without her mother.

This example of a classical repression-based neurosis suggests
that Freud's patients may have been suffering from issues of abandonment as well, but Freud's preoccupation with sexuality blinded
him to other realities. The case of Mrs. Annie Blue Perry demonstrates the importance of a child's dependency on her parents, and
her use of repression to stay attached to her remaining parent serves
as a bridge between Freud's early theory and the explanation for disorders of today.

The Path from Freud's Neurotics to the Disorders That Result in Domestic Violence

Before I describe the intellectual and human path that led from
Freud's early work to our understanding of the dynamics behind
domestic violence, I must define what I mean by *modern disorders.*
Today, most disorders that are seen in outpatient treatment are
defined as *character disorders.* Simply stated, a character or person-

ality disorder is a disorder that is caused by immaturity or malformation of the ego and of the sense of self. These disorders are a consequence of unmet childhood needs that stunt and distort the ego. Adults with character disorders often behave like needy, out-of-control children. Instead of neurotic symptoms, these disorders often involve lack of control of various functions, including eating, drinking, honesty, aggression, sexuality, and/or gambling. The unruly character disorders, taken as a group, are nearly opposite on the dimension of control as compared to neurotic disorders, which are based on overcontrol and often display symptoms that are symbolic of unconscious processes. As we will discover, domestic violence is the consequence of the relationship between two character disorders, one male and one female.

The first two links between the work of Freud and our understanding of the personality disorders of today are the concepts of trauma and repression. Psychological trauma plays an important role in the developmental histories of character disorders; however, the trauma in the histories of these patients occurred in a very different form than the sudden trauma that provoked the neurotic disorders in Freud's day. Most simply, the traumas in the childhoods of now adult character disorders were chronic rather than acute. Their histories are filled with *cumulative traumas,* small undramatic hurts and disappointments that built up year after year, distorting and stunting the individual's ego and devaluing her or his sense of self. Patients with character disorders, like Freud's early neurotic patients, also employ the defense of repression; however, instead of repressing a single traumatic incident as did Katharina, these individuals repress an entire class of painful memories that resulted from years and years of deprivation, abuse, or neglect. The theoretically significant differences between Freud's original model and our understandings today come from the realization that the major source of adult dysfunction is not the conflict between the id and society but rather is the result of the cumulative effects of hundreds of rejections and rebuffs that diminish the developing child's sense of self.

The second important link between Freud's early work and our current understandings of domestic violence is a human rather than a theoretical one. Freud's pioneering work attracted a large number of students and adherents who were dedicated to the proposition that the way to understand an individual's adult problems was to understand the personality structure formed in childhood ("The child is father of the man"). Thus, Freud's method and basic perspective was a starting point for many modifications to his original model that were developed by those who disagreed with one or another part of his theory. One divergent line of thought developed because certain Freudian-trained analysts began studying individuals who were very disturbed but not neurotic. In fact these patients were very different from Freud's neurotics, yet they were analyzed using the same components (id, ego, superego) that Freud used to explain neurosis.

Fairbairn was one such individual, an analyst who had been trained in the classical Freudian school of thought, who then began disagreeing with Freud's theory, even while using Freud's basic method. Fairbairn was one of many theoreticians who began to discover that the dependency of the child on the mother was more important to the development of personality than Freud's belief in the primacy of instinctual drives. One of the disorders that Fairbairn focused on was the "schizoid" disorder, which fifty years ago was known under several different names, including *ambulatory schizophrenia, pseudoneurotic-schizophrenia,* the *"as if" personality,* and the *borderline state* (now called the *borderline personality disorder*). The individuals examined by Fairbairn were more disturbed than the neurotic group studied by Freud but less disturbed than the hallucinating, out-of-contact schizophrenic disorders. Intensive study of this diverse group, again using Freud's original method and concepts, strongly suggested malformation of the ego as the major causative component of the disorder. This discovery was in sharp theoretical contrast to Freud's belief that all problems stemmed from conflict between the id and the constraints of society.

Fairbairn's work had a significant, though indirect, impact on Freud's basic theory. Simply stated, his work, along with that of other theorists in the "English school" of psychoanalysis, began a separate branch of psychoanalytic thought that emphasized the importance of the early relationship between the child and its caretakers with regard to the development of the ego. This school of thought rejected the notion that the id and its sexual motivation was the basis for personality development. Fairbairn's focus on the ego functions of his patients revealed that these individuals had been severely deprived during their development, and that the impoverished relationship with their mothers was the source of their immature and distorted ego structure. In many ways these patients were suffering from inner emptiness, resulting from unmet childhood needs. Classical psychoanalysis had not considered inner emptiness due to poor parenting as either a *symptom* or *cause* of psychological disorders. These psychoanalytically oriented investigators of the English school came to the inescapable conclusion that personality development required that the parent "fill up" the child with positive, nurturing experiences, and that the severe personality disorders they were treating were the result of emotional deprivation due to too little parenting. It was clear that these adult individuals did not have their own internal energy source, but rather suffered from too little mothering during their development. These observations began quietly to challenge the original theory of the primacy of the id. Over time the increased focus on the ego functions of these patients gradually led to the shift of focus in psychoanalytic thinking, away from the "instinctual" demands of the id and toward the developmental demands of the ego. The role of the mother also increased in importance. The reconceptualization of personality disorders by object relations theorists split psychoanalysis into two groups: those who adhered to the original notions regarding the primacy of the concept of the libido, with its biologically motivated drives, and those who abandoned these notions in favor of attachment theory. Classical theory could not survive if it gave up the primary notions of libido and drive, and so the two schools of thought broke apart. The following quotation illustrates the fundamental difference between the classical Freudian position on child development and the position of attachment theory:

> In Freud's view babies are not exploratory beings, open to the world, reaching out with interest and delight towards their mother, capable of love and playfulness, keen to grow and improve their talents. Rather, they begin life in a state of "primary narcissism"; that is, their aim is to turn back to conditions akin to those in the womb; they seek only gratification of their instinctual, physical desires, centered, at this stage, on the mouth, and experience life in terms of an omnipotent fantasy in which the outer world does not exist. Those of us who work in the fields of psychoanalysis or child development have become so accustomed to this concep-

tion—one that is remote from the intuitive experience of mothers—that we often forget how strange and pessimistic it is, and fail
to enquire how Freud got hold of such an absurd notion.
(Lomas 1987:74)

The fact that Freud's theory of child development is now viewed as
absurd did little to help popularize Fairbairn and other object relations theorists of his time, as the mental health establishment was
nearly unanimous in its embrace of Freudian orthodoxy.

Fairbairn's Object Relations Theory

Fairbairn knew of the importance of the mother (the child's
"object") way back in the 1940s, but, as mentioned, his writings
were not influential in the psychoanalytic field during his lifetime.
This was due to the fact that the Second World War was still in
progress, and because there was a second war—a war of opposing
psychoanalytic theories—going on in Great Britain between the two
largest psychoanalytic schools, that of Melanie Klein versus the
school of Anna Freud (Rayner 1991). The English school of psychoanalysis I have already mentioned was actually comprised of three
different schools of thought, each with a different emphasis. The
major conflict was between the theory of Klein, who saw herself as
Freudian loyalist, and Anna Freud. Klein, whose followers were
called the "A" school, believed that the child's innate aggression
was the source of massive ambivalence (love and hate) toward the
mother. Klein was most interested in the effects of primitive
instinctual (id) aggressiveness, which she assumed was the motivating force that impelled the child to keep loving images of the parent split apart from hateful images of the parent in its inner world
(Rayner 1991). Ironically, Klein's line of thought, which emphasized
the activity of the id, influenced others (including Fairbairn) to
expand the concept of *splitting* without relying on the belief in
innate destructiveness of the child. Anna Freud and other analysts
who fled the continent and settled in England just before World War
II comprised the "B" school, which opposed many of the radical
ideas and techniques of Klein. She contributed to object relations
theory by emphasizing and expanding the role of the ego, although
she and her followers retained the concept of the id. Today this

branch of psychoanalysis is called *ego psychology*. There still are analysts strictly allied to Klein's model as well as those who support Anna Freud's position. Neither group, however, could foresee the influence that *parts* of their model, when combined, would exert on the entire field.

Fairbairn belonged to the loosely organized "independent" school of psychoanalytic theorists, independent of both Melanie Klein and Anna Freud, with few followers of his own. His position was largely ignored by the two English rivals, and completely ignored by the larger classical school of thought. It remained dormant until America was introduced to the borderline personality disorder in 1966, when one analyst, Otto Kernberg, integrated the prior work of Fairbairn, Klein, and other independent-school theorists into a comprehensive "new" model of the borderline personality disorder. Kernberg's introduction of these concepts to the American mental health community unleashed a flood of books on the topic. Today, object relations theory is still composed of small separate factions that disagree on various issues. However, most of the current literature takes the many contributions of analytic writers who were interested in the effects of the early interpersonal environment on the development of the child's ego structure and merges them conceptually to form object relations theory. Overall, it has more adherents than classical psychoanalysis, from which it developed.

The Object and the Developing Child's Need for Attachment

Perhaps the worst and least descriptive word in the field of modern psychological theories is *object*, which is defined as a person outside of the self. Originally Freud assumed that the child was attracted to the mother because she was a "sexual object" that allowed him or her to discharge pent up sexualized or other instinctual drives such as hunger, thirst, or irritation due to discharge of wastes. One has to remember that, to Freud, all human motivation, including the newborn's desire to nurse at its mother's breast was sexualized motivation. Therefore, persons outside the infant were all assumed to be sexualized objects. With the trend toward object relations theory the notion that sexual motivation underlies all human behavior has been reduced, but, sadly, not the use of the word *object* to denote a person other than the infant. Therefore, an object is anyone but ourselves—we are all objects to each other.

Fairbairn clearly saw that Freud's concept of human development, based on biological energies that moved from place to place in the body, was archaic. In fact, Fairbairn once stated that Freud's libido theory was acting like a "brake" on the wheel of progress. This was not a diplomatic statement to make in the 1940s, since it alienated many of the traditionalists in his limited audience, all of whom were trained in the Freudian model.

Fairbairn was sure of his own model because he worked with abandoned and abused children in foundling homes, unlike Freud, who worked with neurotic adults. He got to see firsthand the fundamental and indivisible source of human motivation in these distressed children. Fairbairn recognized that the bottom line of human motivation was not sexualized drives but the absolute need of these children to be connected to their mothers. The attachment between mother and infant was absolutely essential for survival, because it gave the child both psychological and physiological life. He observed the extreme terror and emotional collapse experienced by abused and abandoned children when they were placed in the foundling home, despite the fact that the foundling home provided them with safety from further physical abuse by their parents. Many of these children who were forcibly separated from their abusive parents behaved as if they felt they were going to die—even though continued association with their violent and dangerous parents would itself have been life threatening to them. Amazingly, these children preferred to face the threat of being *beaten to death in their own homes by their own parents rather than the physical safety of staying in the foundling home without their parents.* In order to illustrate this counterintitutive point Fairbairn once invited Harry Guntrip, another psychoanalytic theorist, to the foundling home to demonstrate the deep attachment that abused children have toward their violent and dangerous parents. He asked an eight-year-old girl (who had been removed from her home by the authorities in Edinburgh, Scotland, because her mother had beaten her cruelly) if she would like him to find her a good, brand-new mother. The young girl recoiled in horror and insisted that she wanted her own violent and physically abusive mother back (Guntrip 1975:146).

Fairbairn's model of personality development had at its center the attachment between mother and child. The quality and characteristics of this first relationship, the satisfaction or frustration of the child's developmental needs were for Fairbairn the key factors that influenced the development of the child's personality. Fairbairn's model is commonsensical and many readers will recognize many of his positions as those that have moved into the mainstream of our thinking today. His first point was that the greatest trauma that children can suffer is to feel fundamentally unloved by their mothers. Not only does the child need to feel loved, but the love that she returns to her mother needs to be accepted as valuable. If this is not the case the child will experience herself, and her love, as worthless, and eventually keep all expressions of it inside. This position is completely acceptable today, but when Fairbairn wrote in 1940 the whole mental health world was convinced that sexual traumas, oedipal conflicts, and other such dramatic issues governed human development.

Fairbairn then noticed, again from his direct observation of mothers and infants, that the young child was intensely focused on one person and one person only. He recognized that infants and young children do not have the same freedom to choose different objects that the adult has. In fact, the focus on the single object (the mother or caretaker) is intense, and unfamiliar people frighten the young child. Anyone who has seen a lost child in a supermarket can attest to the fact that he is not interested in candy or the store manager or anyone else but his mother. In fact, "kindly" people who approach a lost child only make him more distressed. Fairbairn recognized from this observation that the child's dependency on his object—whether it be a mature nurturing mother or an alcoholic and physically abusing mother—is absolute.

The Paradoxical Consequence of Early Rejection

The next two points that Fairbairn made are not as apparent but follow inexorably when any child is rejected by his all-important parent. The first is that the rejected child is *more* rather than less attached to his mother than is the loved and accepted child. How can this be? Common sense would suggest that the rejected child should be *less* attached because of the experience of constant rejection. This incorrect but logical notion is based on the assumption that the child has the same freedom of choice that adults do. Fairbairn had already recognized that the child had no choice whatever to reject her parent. She is simply stuck, and has to accept the parent, regardless of how poorly the parent behaves toward her. Whatever nurturance and support the mother does not provide will not be forgotten, but it will conversely be longed for by the child, and, later, by the developing adolescent until the unmet need is satisfied. Young children, including abused and neglected ones, are absolutely *fixated* (to use a Freudian term somewhat improperly) on their mothers. The more they are deprived, the more they are fixated.

Fairbairn saw that the child's "choice" (rejecting or accepting her mother) was one of choosing life or death. In other words, there was no choice for the child. To illustrate this point, he described a dream of one of his severely disturbed adult patients. The patient dreamt that he was a starving child, and went into his mother's room where she was sleeping. There was a bowl of his favorite dessert, chocolate pudding, next to her on the nightstand, but he shuddered to realize that it contained poison. He knew that if he did not eat the pudding he would die of starvation, but if he did he would get sick and die of the poison. This patient then reported that he ate the pudding in his dream and became terribly ill. This is Fairbairn's point—the neglected or abused child has no options whatever. The child is never able to protect himself from the "poison" because he has such pressing needs; whatever the parent gives him, no matter how damaging it is, is what he gets. The child is so focused on the object, pressured by intense needs that cannot be denied, that he is completely unable to protect himself from accepting harmful forms of abuse from his objects. His attachment to his needed object *will destroy him* but he has no choice in the matter, because his need for the mother is absolute.

As time goes on the rejected child needs *more* rather than *less* support. For instance, the consistently deprived five-year-old child requires not only that his five-year-old needs be met, but also the neglected needs from when he was four, and those from when he was three, and so on. The pattern is reversed for the normally reared child who, as she develops, can sustain herself on less and less parental support. I once wrote a report for a puzzled staff of a prison for "youthful" offenders. I was asked to explain why one of the most vicious and violent fourteen-year-old inmates that they had ever seen was repeatedly observed sucking his thumb and rocking himself to sleep clutching a teddy bear. This young man had repeatedly sexually molested his two nieces when they were left in his care. The "behavioral" explanation (based on the stimulus-reinforcement model) for this behavior offered by the staff was that this inmate got attention from them when he displayed thumb sucking. These behaviorally trained professionals were puzzled by the unlikely (to their way of thinking) juxtaposition of violence and infantile neediness in the same person. This violent and aggressive young man demonstrated the needs left from his early deprivation, which seemed out of place since they existed in a person who also displayed the violence of an "adult." As we will see, when we examine male batterers, the lack of emotional support during childhood does not go away, but instead shows up in later years. Indeed, one of the most frequent responses to lack of early nurturance in males is rage and destructiveness that is projected outward toward weaker "others." Violence is often assumed to be an adult behavior, however, it is often the consequence of poorly understood infantile needs that emerge in a person with an adult body who is paradoxically driven by the needs of an infant.

Learning Theory and The Behavioristic Model

The last psychological model that is in the competition to explain why battered women return to the men who abuse them had a very different, and independent, beginning. Behaviorism began in Germany in the latter half of the nineteenth century. A number of early scientists began studying human perception under laboratory conditions. They originally investigated the amount that any given stimulus had to be increased before change could be perceived by the human subject. For instance, how much lighter did a one-ounce weight have to be before the subject could reliably say it was lighter than another actual one-ounce weight? This amount was called a *JND*, a just noticeable difference. The approach emphasized careful "scientific" study based on controlled conditions, measurable stimuli, and repeatability. That is, the interested American psychologist could read a paper on the study of "just noticeable differences" in weight stimuli done in Germany and confirm it with a study performed under the same conditions in America.

The scientific study of human characteristics moved from the earliest investigation of perception to the study of learning and conditioning. Nearly every undergraduate student in psychology is familiar with the famous (and somewhat sadistic) experiment conducted by John Watson in 1920. He and a colleague first exposed their nine-month-old subject, Albert B., to a variety of animals (a white rat, a rabbit, and a dog) to see if he had any natural fear responses. Albert displayed no signs of fear and two months later they reintroduced the white rat and banged a steel bar behind Albert's head the moment he reached toward the rat. The loud noise frightened Albert considerably, and he developed a conditioned emotional response (fear) to the presence of the rat. Then Watson retested Albert with different animals to see if the fear generalized from the rat to other similar animals. Others looked at different forms of conditioning. The Russian laboratories of Pavlov conditioned dogs to salivate to a bell. Pavlov began by squirting meat powder into the dog's mouth when the bell rang. After a number of such experiences the dog would salivate to the sound of the bell, even if there was no meat powder. Pavlov's conditioning was called *classical* conditioning.

Over time, Watson and, later, B. F. Skinner developed a body of literature on operant conditioning that presented itself as a viable model of human development. The learning or behavioral model provides a coherent model of language and skill acquisition and assumes that all behaviors can be broken down into sequences of stimulus and reinforcement. Like Freudian theory, which learning theorists passionately despise for being unscientific, learning theory reduces humankind not to sexual drives, as did Freud, but to learners of reinforced (or punishing) sequences. Learning theory is most useful in the field of training, and in the therapy of specific limited symptoms such as isolated phobias. It strongly objects to any model that produces hypotheses about internal dynamics (such as the existence of a sense of self) because these inferred processes cannot be directly measured or observed. Learning theory is reviewed here because it has been used to explain adult attachments to hurtful parents/lovers/friends. Lenore Walker, in her book *The Battered Woman*, cites a specific type of learning called "learned helplessness" as the explanation for the battered woman's inability to escape from the batterer. I will examine the ability of learning theory to explain the return of the abused woman to her battering partner in chapter 5.

Summary

This chapter has covered much material, from the concept of a psychological model, to the history and evolution of object relations theory, to Fairbairn's theory of personality development, and, finally, to the behavioral model of human development. I began with Freud and his instinctual theory because of the theoretical and human links with object relations theory, and because many of Freud's concepts, including repression and the unconscious, are carried over in Fairbairn's model and have withstood the test of time.

I presented Fairbairn's model because it explains the underlying personality structure of those individuals who eventually find themselves involved in domestic abuse, either as the perpetrator or as the victim. Fairbairn observed that children are completely and utterly dependent upon their caretakers. His model shifted the focus of study away from the Freudian concepts of psychosexual development to the study of the quality and style of attachment between mother and infant. Fairbairn recognized that the greatest trauma that a child could experience was not to be loved by a mother. He also recognized that the infant is focused on one parent as the source of all love and nurturance. His most important contribution was his observation that the rejected child was *more* rather than *less* attached to the frustrating mother. The increase in the child's attachment was due to the fact that her or his needs were being ignored, needs that absolutely had to be met by that one and only parent. Similarly, Fairbairn observed that his abused children preferred to return to their abusive homes, and risk suffering more grievous injuries, rather than remaining in the safety of the foundling home. The following chapters will build on Fairbairn's original contributions until the reader has a complete model of the inner world of the abuser and his victim.

CHAPTER TWO

The Three Basic
Ego Processes
That Lead to
Psychological Maturity

In this chapter I will review the development of the human ego structure. The material in this section is not based specifically on Fairbairn's work, rather it is from two related fields of thought: ego psychology, which is a subset of psychoanalytic thought that focuses on the development of the infant's ego capacities, and attachment theory, which originated with the work of John Bowlby. Attachment theory is rooted in ethnology, the study of human and animal behavior in the natural environment. Bowlby was inspired by the early work of Konrad Lorenz, who had observed that ducklings developed a strong bond with the mother duck, despite the fact that they were never fed by her. Ducklings find their own food from birth and therefore "drive" theory cannot explain the bond to their mother because there is no drive reduction (feeding) involved in the mother duck's parenting behavior. Bowlby investigated the bond between human parents and their children from ethnology's theory-free perspective, and developed the model now called attachment theory. Both ego psychology and attachment theory will be used throughout this chapter as they give slightly different, but compatible interpretations to various aspects of the mother-child relationship.

Attachment theory looks at the healthy and adaptive nature of careseeking, thus removing the pejorative stigma of the concept of dependency:

> Attachment theory regards the propensity to make intimate emotional bonds to particular individuals as a basic component of

human nature, already present in germinal form in the neonate and continuing through adult life into old age. During infancy and childhood bonds are with parents (or parent substitutes) who are looked to for protection, comfort and support. . . . Within the attachment framework therefore intimate emotional bonds are seen as neither subordinate to nor derivative from food and sex. Nor is the urgent desire for comfort and support in adversity regarded as childish, as dependency theory implies. Instead the capacity to make intimate emotional bonds with other individuals, sometimes in the careseeking role and sometimes in the caregiving one, is regarded as a principal feature of effective personality functioning and mental health. (Bowlby 1988:120–121)

In this quote Bowlby clearly differentiates his theoretical position both from Freudian theory and from ego psychology. He notes that emotional attachment to others is not a lesser human trait than the need for food or sex, and that it is not a consequence of these needs but rather an innate and equally powerful need in itself. Further, he points out that the pursuit of comfort of individuals of any age is not a pathological but rather a normal behavior. The great strength of attachment theory is that it has generated volumes of empirical research about mother-infant interactions and the effects of early deprivation on later behavior.

For example, Bowlby has observed that there is a predictable pattern to mother-infant interactions, involving an onset, followed by intense engagement, and terminating with the infant's withdrawal when she becomes sated. This is often followed by another cycle of greeting, interaction, and withdrawal. Bowlby observed that the cycle is determined by the child's spontaneous needs rather than by the mother's needs, and that the sensitive mother regulated her behavior so that it meshed with the infant:

What emerges from these studies is that the ordinary sensitive mother is quickly attuned to her infant's natural rhythms and, by attending to the details of his behavior, discovers what suits him and behaves accordingly. By so doing she not only makes him contented but also enlists his co-operation. (Bowlby 1988:9)

Bowlby also reported an impressive study of maternal sensitivity done by Ainsworth (1977) in which raters visited a group of twenty-three mothers and infants in their homes for a three-hour observation and rating session. These observations were recorded on four nine-point scales, one of which rated the mother's sensitivity to the infant's signals and communications. These long rating sessions were done every three weeks for the first year of the infant's life. Then these children were tested at one year of age in a "slightly strange situation," an empty room with a single large toy in it. The infants were rated as to how active they were in their exploration of the strange situation and how they reacted to their mothers presence, her departure and her return. The twenty-three children behaved in ways that placed them into three distinct groups that were labeled X, Y, and Z. The X group consisted of eight children who were deemed securely attached, in that they were active, interacted easily with their mother, and greeted her warmly when she returned. The Z group (containing eleven of the twenty-three subjects) displayed a very different pattern of behavior, as described by Bowlby:

> Three of them were passive, both at home and in the test situation; they explored little and, instead, sucked a thumb or rocked. Constantly anxious about mother's whereabouts, they cried much in her absence but were contrary and difficult on her return. The other eight in this group alternated between appearing very independent and ignoring mother altogether, and then suddenly becoming anxious and trying to find her. Yet, when they did find her, they seemed not to enjoy contact with her, and often they struggled to get away again. (Bowlby 1988:47)

These anxious, fearful, and ambivalent children in this group had mothers who were rated lowest on the rating scale of maternal attentiveness. Conversely, the nonanxious X group of eight children had mothers who were rated highest in terms of responsivity to their infants' needs. The Y group was in between, both in terms of ratings in the strange situation and in terms of the ratings of their mothers' attentiveness at home. This is exactly what one would expect, and it strongly contradicts the Freudian position that the mother's behavior is not influential on the child's psychological development.

How did the mothers of the Z group become so unresponsive to their infants' needs? Other studies done by researchers on attachment theory offer answers to this question. Research has demonstrated that high levels of sensitivity to their infant's needs are absent in mothers who were separated prematurely from one or both of their parents before the age of eleven. These mothers were observed in their own homes and compared to young mothers with normal histories. The mothers from poorer family histories interacted significantly less with their infants in that they were out of sight of their infants, on average, for twice as long as the control group. Even when interacting with their infants these mothers spent less time, on average, holding, looking at, and talking to them when compared to the control group. Bowlby cites this study done by Wolkind, Hall, and Pawlby (1977), to demonstrate the generational effect of inadequate parenting on the following generation. These mothers were less attached, less concerned, and less attuned to their infants because of their own histories of flawed parenting.

Ego Psychology's Approach to the Development of the Personality

Ego psychology is, as previously mentioned, a cousin to object relations theory, and evolved from Anna Freud's work, which emphasized the role of the ego in child development. It differs from object relations theory in that it still assumes that the id is the source of energy for the personality. This model focuses on the role of the three fundamental processes that contribute to the maturation of the child's ego: differentiation, integration, and introjection. Each of these impressively labeled processes will be examined in some detail. In simplest terms *differentiation* refers to the infant's dawning realization that she is separate from her mother. The culmination of a healthy course of differentiation is the emergence of a uniquely "new" individual rather than a clone of her parents. The term *integration* refers to the ability of the developing child to gradually understand that she has but one mother, not two separate ones. Prior to the achievement of integration the infant assumes that she has one good (gratifying) mother and another, completely separate, bad (rejecting) mother. A healthy course of integration culminates in an adult who views others as whole persons, one who doesn't lose sight of a person's goodness, even when that individual is temporarily angry at him. The third developmental process of the ego is called *introjection*; it refers to the internalization of memories of being cared for (or of being rejected) that build up inside the child and either support her during times of stress or undermine her sense of self later in life. Positive memories lead to the inner strength that we often call "good character." Introjection occurs simultaneously and concurrently with differentiation and integration.

Differentiation: The First Developmental Process

Differentiation will be discussed first because it is the first of the three process that can be observed during the child's development. Introjection occurs at the same time; however, it cannot be observed at the early stages of life. The concept of differentiation actually has two closely related meanings: one refers to differentiation of the self from other persons; the other refers to differentiation within the self. Differentiation of self from others is defined as a person's ability to experience him or herself as existing and operating separately from others in the human environment. When used in this manner differentiation refers first to the overall awareness of the infant that its mother and itself are separate entities. This awareness sounds ridiculously simple, but, as we will see, there are many who do not fully achieve this fundamental understanding.

The second way that the concept of differentiation is used focuses on the individual's self, and it refers to the ability to identify one subtle feeling state as being different from another. Let me illustrate by using wine tasting as a simple analogy for the individual's development of the ability to differentiate among many subtle internal feeling states in his interior world. The beginning wine taster may be unable to tell two glasses apart; perhaps the only distinction possible is red from white or sweet from sour. Later the increasingly sophisticated taster will be able to identify Bordeaux wines from those wines grown in Burgundy as well as wines from California. The more experienced the wine taster becomes, the greater her ability will be to differentiate one subtle taste from another. Ultimately, the most sophisticated tasters are able to distinguish one year's growth from lesser or better vintages of the same vineyard. The same holds true for the human ability to gradually differentiate among subtle differences in the feeling states within one's interior world.

The human infant at birth is undifferentiated in every sense of the word. Not only is she unaware that she is a separate human being from her mother, but she cannot differentiate one feeling from the next. The following dramatic quote from Margaret Little, an English psychoanalyst and theorist (actually describing adults who regressed back to an undifferentiated childlike state) illustrates the experience of an extreme lack of differentiation:

> Tension is experienced as something intolerable, threatening life itself. . . . That is to say there is only a *state of being* or of experiencing and no sense of there being a person. There is only an anger, fear, love, movement, etc., but no person *feeling* anger, fear, or love, or moving. And since all these things are one and the same, there is no separateness or distinction between them.
>
> (Little 1981:84)

Into this confused, disorganized chaos comes the caretaker, usually the mother, whose task is to meet her infant's overwhelming needs. It is the caretaker's attunement to the distressed infant's needs that turns frightening, unendurable tension into satisfaction and contentment. The mother's calm and appropriate reactions to the infant's distress gradually teaches the infant that there are separate sources of tension, and, more important, that "others" can be trusted and relied upon to relieve distress.

D. W. Winnicott (1986), another British object relations theorist of Fairbairn's era, worked as a pediatrician before focusing on psychoanalytic theory. He observed that skillful mothers had the ability to understand the needs of their children—even before they developed language. Often the skilled mother has to use her sensitivity to her infant's needs to "diagnose" her toddler's distress and determine whether hunger, tiredness, or fear of separation is the problem. He called this heightened sensitivity of mothers to the needs of their infants *primary maternal preoccupation.*

The accurate responsivity of the skilled mother, whom Winnicott called the "good enough mother," helps the infant make sense of her own inner experience. For instance, the newborn does not know the source of tension that is making her cry. The mother's responsiveness, and accurate analysis of her infant's needs, begins to link needs together with maternal responses in the child's mind. The well-cared-for child experiences the world as a place that is responsive to her needs, a place where her needs are seen as important, and a place where she is protected. The attentiveness of the mother to the child's needs, and the increased level of meaningfulness of their communications, gradually allows the child to develop accurate methods of understanding what she feels. The clear and helpful responses of the caretaker aid the developing infant to distinguish a particular source of tension. With the development of language the good enough mother can question the child and find out what the source of tension is, thus furthering the differentiation of one internal state from others. If, on the other hand, the mother constantly misinterprets the child's signals, then there is going to be an enormous lack of understanding within that child as to the existence of separate and distinct internal tensions, as well as a huge reservoir of unmet needs. For instance, one patient remembered that her mother had one "solution" for all of her various tensions, which was to feed her, no matter what the problem.

The Research of Margaret Mahler's on Stages of Separation and Individuation

Before I turn to the other two ego developmental processes, (introjection and integration), I want to describe the research from the ego psychology perspective on the process of differentiation carried out by Margaret Mahler and her colleagues (Mahler, Pine, and Bergman 1975). The model that Mahler developed is very tied to laboratory observations, which makes it empirical rather than purely theoretical. Her stages of psychological individuation are used as the ego development model for most object relations theories. Mahler and her colleagues carefully studied mothers and infants, and developed a series of descriptions of the normal stages that a child goes through during differentiation.

Surprisingly, differentiation from the mother does not begin immediately at birth. First, there is a stage that Mahler called *symbiosis*, which lasts until approximately nine months and is characterized by extreme psychological closeness between mother and infant. During this stage the infant shows no signs that she experiences her mother as a separate person. In fact, this is a period of time during which there is a "dual unity" between the infant's nascent ego and her mother. There is no "ego boundary" between infant and mother, and feelings flow freely back and forth between them. Anxiety in the mother is instantly conveyed to the infant, who can do nothing to protect herself from the mother's distress. Conversely, the distressed infant causes reciprocal anxiety in her mother. The mother's physical touch, smile, and responses give the child its earliest sense of itself as a living being. During a normal period of symbiosis the infant becomes deeply attached to her mother; this early attachment and trust widens later in life to include others.

Clearly, separation from the good enough mother during symbiosis, or indifferent parenting by a preoccupied or disturbed mother, can lead to disastrous consequences for the developing child. For instance, one former patient of mine related to others "robotically." He was a brilliant engineer who was sent all over the world troubleshooting electronic problems in military aircraft. Even in the world of the military his colleagues found him to be cold, aloof, and impervious to the feelings of others. In therapy, which he approached with the same mechanical intensity and coolness, he remembered a story that his family had repeated a number of times about what a "good" baby he had been. His mother was a depressed, highly religious woman, who had had three children in quick succession, the last being my patient. She soon realized that this baby seemed unfussy and content, and she left him alone for long periods of time in his crib while she attended to the incessant needs of her two older, more demanding children. Soon this isolated and ignored infant became mute and unresponsive, staring into space. This aroused the anxiety of his father, a state trooper, who ordinarily paid no attention to his children at all. He became so concerned about his youngest son's unresponsiveness that he would stop home every day and take him out of the crib and attempt to play with him. At some level this ordinarily incompetent father saw the damage that was being done to his son, and he tried to compensate for the neglect.

The first stage of differentiation begins as symbiosis wanes, at about nine months of age, and is characterized by the infant's exploration of the mother's body, which indicates that he sees her as a separate person. For instance, the infant will no longer mold himself to the mother and instead might arch away so he can look at his mother's face. He might reach up and touch or pull his mother's nose, thus indicating that he is aware of a person outside himself. This first stage of separation is followed by a second, more active phase, which was called "practicing" by Mahler and her associates. This stage is characterized by the physical development of muscles and coordination, which allows the child first to crawl and then walk by himself. This stage is characterized by exuberant exploration of the world. The child's success during this stage depends upon the success of the earlier stages. If, for instance, the child had been neglected during symbiosis, then his exploration of the world will be impaired, as he will have to stay very close to his mother for fear of losing her. Conversely, those toddlers with good enough early histories will rely on their memories from the symbiotic and the first differentiation stages to "fuel" them during their explorations.

The "terrible twos" is the commonly used term to describe the third phase of separation, which Mahler called *rapprochement*. This is a conflict-laden stage of development, because the child is more aware of separateness from his mother. During the previous practicing phase the younger child was unaware of her separateness, and so her eager legs could take her through the house with great exuberance. Now, the two-year-old is physically capable of going further, but her separation from her caretaker is more obvious to her, and this awareness produces anxiety. Simultaneously, the developing child is pushed by increasing needs for autonomy, and so the clash between the desire to separate and the opposite fear of getting lost provokes a great deal of conflict. One moment the child may want to be on her own, while the next she might demand that mother stay right next to her. These sudden alterations can bewilder the most patient parent.

The final phase of differentiation and individuation begins after rapprochement has run its course, perhaps at around thirty-six months. This is an open-ended stage where the second major ego development process, integration, begins. During this period the child is gradually able to integrate or merge the separate views of her mother into a single view and, reciprocally, is able to hold a single view of herself as well. The process of integration will be discussed later in this chapter.

Differentiation both from external objects and within the interior world does not end suddenly but rather continues through young adulthood. For instance, the six-year-old mimics every opinion of his parents, the twelve-year-old may have some opinions from his peers thrown into the mix, while the eighteen-year-old in her first year of college may exaggerate her separateness from her conservative businesswoman mother by spouting Marx. It is not just opinions that indicate increasing differentiation but also a growing independent and stable sense of self that is not easily influenced by others. A well-differentiated young adult is able to resist the influence of anyone, including parents, if it appears that the result of the influence will cause them harm.

Lack of Differentiation in Adulthood

Growing up does not guarantee increased differentiation, and many chronological adults can, and do, relate to their parents or others in a poorly differentiated manner. Adults who were unable to differentiate from their mothers during childhood are unable to function independently in adulthood, or, if they are forced to, they will experience extreme anxiety. The following example illustrates an acute lack of differentiation in thirty-seven-year-old twins:

> Greta and Freda Chapin, 37, are identical twins who dress alike, walk in step, take two-hour baths together and frequently talk— and sometimes swear—in unison. If separated, even for a moment, they wail and scream. . . . The Chapins wear identical gray coats, but one originally came with green buttons, and the other with gray. So they cut two buttons off each, and now both coats have two green and two gray. . . . A social worker once gave them two bars of different colored soap, and they burst into tears. Then they cut the bars in half so they each had the same. (Leo 1981:45)

This terribly sad example illustrates just how severe lack of differentiation can be in chronological adults. These twins experienced acute anxiety the moment they were separated, either physically or symbolically, somewhat like a young infant separated from his mother. Separation produced severe anxiety because the sense of self inside each of these twins was so empty that it could not sustain either individual when apart. This example illustrates how severe the problem can be; however most patients display less dramatic forms of lack of differentiation, as the following example shows:

> Cathy came in for therapy with a whole series of problems revolving around her mother's interference and intrusiveness into her life. She was a divorced mother of a five-year-old son and had moved back into her parents' home to save money, despite the fact that she had ample income won in her divorce and a full-time job. She and her mother would bicker constantly over child raising

issues, and Cathy felt (rightly so) that her mother was trying to take over the rearing of her child. She worked as a receptionist at a dental office and was constantly harassed by calls from her mother during the day. During these intense, emotionally laden calls, her mother might insist that Cathy "take back" something she had said the night before, or she might inform Cathy that she had rearranged her furniture in a way that Cathy had opposed. Despite the apparent strife and conflict between them, Cathy was "afraid" to hang up the phone on her mother. In fact, when her mother failed to call her every two hours, Cathy would call home, fearful that something had happened to her mother. Cathy and her mother would fight if they discovered they had different opinions about any given topic, because even minor differences of opinion made one or the other feel abandoned and isolated. After her first therapy session with me, Cathy ran home and told her mother everything that I said about her situation.

Lack of differentiation is a key to understanding both males and females who desperately return to destructive relationships. Cathy, in this example, reported that she was afraid to hang up the phone on her mother. Her fear was not a fabrication, since she unconsciously recognized that without her mother there would be no possibility of ever "making up" the nurturing that she had missed out on while she was growing up. Fairbairn noted that the fundamental reason the underloved and undersupported child cannot leave the parent is because separation from that parent would end all hope of ever receiving the support and nurturing that he/she still required. This is one of the principal reasons for what Fairbairn originally called the "return to the bad object."

Adults with poor developmental histories also seek out and remain in undifferentiated relationships because it makes them feel less empty and alone. Undifferentiated relationships allow the external person, in this case Cathy's mother, to partially "penetrate into" the sense of self of the other person; her daughter. Cathy's mother was constantly fighting to get in Cathy's inner world and take her over. This apparent struggle has an unconscious payoff in that it temporarily saves both participants from feeling abandoned. That is, both Cathy and her mother felt less alone when they sensed that they were extremely close, almost as if they were the same person. This feeling of undifferentiated closeness reduces the sense of emptiness and abandonment that stalks those individuals with poor early histories. Thus, both Cathy and her mother experienced some sense of relief from their inner emptiness due to their undifferentiated relationship.

Undifferentiated adult relationships are often called "merged," "enmeshed," or "engulfed" relationships. The normal healthy sense of self has a firm boundary around it that cannot be breached. The empty, emotionally abandoned, individual invites others "on the outside" to come "inside," in order to make them feel whole. The reader can see that several injustices had been done to Cathy by her mother. First, her mother deprived her of the necessary nurturing that would have allowed her to differentiate normally. She did not deprive her daughter out of malice, but rather because she had never received proper parenting herself and thus had nothing to give the next generation. Then she used her daughter as a defense against her own emptiness, and Cathy complied, for she was empty too and felt better when her mother was psychologically "with" her.

Lack of differentiation between the adult partners is the most commonly seen characteristic in couples engaged in the battering scenario. It is mutual in that both the batterer and his abused partner are poorly differentiated from each other. I once worked with an abused woman who managed to separate from her husband briefly. Her husband was so primitively enraged by this rejection that he returned to their home with a rifle and shot holes through the front door, while she and her two children were inside. He was arrested and jailed, however upon his release they were reunited, and she began coming to my office for weekly therapy sessions. During her sessions, he would remain parked outside the building with both children in the car and with the engine running, waiting for her to emerge. My patient was as desperately dependent and undifferentiated from her husband as he was from her. When they were together, their separate senses of self merged together and gave each of them enough sense of safety and wholeness to function. When she was alone my patient was unable to leave her house, yet in our therapy sessions she said that she hated her husband with a deep and abiding passion. This paradoxical combination of extreme dependency, lack of differentiation and mutual hostility will be discussed again in chapter 5.

Parental Behaviors That Interfere With the Child's Differentiation From Objects

Healthy mothers understand that by supporting a child's developmental achievements they are paving the way for that child's ultimate independence. Sadly, many mothers unconsciously cannot tolerate the child's increased separation during development because the child's love has been used to support the parent's empty sense of self. Many of these mothers have experienced severely impoverished histories with their own parents and have poor adult relationships as well. They rely on their intense connectedness with their children for their entire emotional sustenance. These immature parents see the world as an enormously frightening place, and their children become the only persons they feel they can depend upon for love and comfort. A number of mothers have told me that they conceived children for the sole purpose of fulfilling their need to be loved. It is paradoxical that these adult women were motivated to become a mothers by their pressing unmet childhood needs, and nothing suited their purposes better than an infant of their very own. The unfortunate child who is born to a parent with these needs is forced into the role of "captive audience," one who is expected to supply his or her mother with all the love that she did not receive from her own parents.

In a similar vein, other fragile mothers have said that they assumed that their two-year-old toddlers "hate" them when they willfully run from them during the practicing stage of development. These insecure mothers are ignorant of the normal stages of child development and rely on their toddler's dependency on them to support their fragile sense of worth. If the child develops and separates, then the personal worth of these mothers can collapse. This is a dangerous situation for the unknowing infant because his normal strivings for autonomy and separation are opposed by his mother and she cannot support them. This point has been made by Bowlby, who also cites a secondary, defense-based damage that results from the child's need to deny the destructive aspects of his relationship with his mother:

> One such is when a mother, who herself had a childhood deprived of love, seeks from her own child the love she has hitherto lacked. In doing this she is inverting the normal parent-child relationship,

requiring the child to act as parent whilst she becomes a child. To someone unaware of what is going on it may appear that the child is being "overindulged," but a closer look shows that mother is placing a heavy burden on him. What is of special relevance here is that more often than not the child is expected to be grateful for such care as he receives and not to notice the demands being made upon him. One result of this is that, in conformity with his mother's wishes, he builds up a one-sided picture of her as wholly loving and generous, thereby shutting away from conscious processing much information also reaching him that she is often selfish, demanding and ungrateful. (Bowlby 1988:107)

Thus the engulfed child is damaged in two separate ways. First, his normal autonomy needs for exploration, the development of new skills, and expanded relationships with peers are thwarted. Second, he learns to repress the reality that his mother is a self-centered woman who is using his imposed dependency for her own gratification. He learns to deny a substantial aspect of reality, and the denial of parental failure is one of the most common characteristics of of the neglected or engulfed child.

There is a third *extremely* negative consequence to a child that is due to his mother's inability to differentiate from him, and that is the child's inability to develop normal and expectable control of his behavior. The poorly differentiated mother cannot discipline her child, because the child's distress when he is being disciplined "feels" like overwhelming distress *to her*. The lack of an appropriate ego boundary between them allows the child's anger and frustration when he is disciplined to pour directly back into his mother's consciousness. Amazingly, *these mothers feel like they themselves are being punished when they try to discipline their own children*. They can't tolerate the child's distress and soon give up all attempts at appropriate discipline. Instead, they often try to control their increasingly unmanageable children with bribery or with various forms of indulgence. This is also determined by their impoverished histories and lack of differentiation—when these parents indulge their children they themselves feel vicariously gratified, and this makes up for some of the constant emptiness they feel. This is a tragic situation for the child because he is not able to achieve the necessary discipline to function outside the dysfunctional home. For instance, when the child who has been "reared" in this type of environment reaches school, his lack of self-control will prove an immediate problem for the teachers. He will not be able to interact cooperatively with the other children and will not tolerate any form of punishment of his self-centered behaviors. If the child is in any way censured by the school, these fragile mothers will typically attack the school personnel ferociously, since they feel personally attacked, again because their child is experienced as being part of themselves.

James Masterson (1988) studied the families of poorly differentiated adolescents and reported that there was an easily identifiable pattern within dysfunctional families that allowed the mothers of his young patients to continue an undifferentiated relationship with the child, while the fathers withdrew:

> The specifics vary from family to family, but in general the father of the borderline child does not intrude on the mother-child relationship. His influence is almost always, by default, a reinforcement of the mother-child's exclusive clinging relationship, rather than as a force to oppose it by leading the child away into the broader world. . . . I discovered that an unconscious emotional contract, most often never verbalized, had existed between the couples in which the mother allowed the father to distance himself from the home for whatever reason or interest, be it career, hobby, or other friendships, in exchange for the mother's getting the exclusive right to care for—and control—the child. . . . What I learned was that the mother didn't want the father at home, especially if he sought to play the normal role of a "rescuer" or savior to take the child out of her control and introduce the child to the larger reality. (Masterson 1988:56–57)

Mothers are the child-rearing "agents" of our society. They do not act in faulty ways toward their children because of malice. As we also see from Masterson's research, they do not act alone, but often have a compliant husband whose own personality defects abet the destruction of the next generation. Caregivers in general, and mothers in particular, are formed by the values of the culture in which they are raised, and reflect the strengths and weaknesses of that culture. In this culture we still value men's achievements over women's, pay men higher wages than women in equivalent jobs, and generally value men's opinions more highly than women's. Child rearing is often performed by individuals who feel demeaned, have little power compared to their male counterparts, and have suffered from being raised by mothers who were themselves ill prepared to nurture their offspring, male or female. All these negative trends funnel into many of our mothers, who are then naively expected by our society to produce healthy, self assured, confident, and high-functioning children.

Introjection: A Parallel Developmental Process of the Ego

Introjection is the second major developmental process of the ego, and it occurs simultaneously and in parallel with differentiation, although, unlike differentiation, it is not an obvious process. While introjection begins at the first moment of life, the images and memories that the child internalizes are vague and poorly categorized in the very young infant's mind. The internalization, categorization, and retrieval of memories of love and care (or of frustration and neglect)—memories that are based on prior interactions with the caregiver(s)—comprise this ego developmental process. Positive memories serve as the fuel that allows the child to separate physically and emotionally from her objects, and, in adulthood, gives the individual a sense of personal strength. We already know that *object* refers to a person outside the self. Memories of external objects become internalized or *introjected* when the child is able to remember the characteristics of her parents even if they are not physically present. These internalized objects are made of packages or groupings of emotionally similar memories of events that actually took place in relation to the parents. For instance, the child groups together memories of being cared for by the mother into a single "good mother" internal image. These groupings become more detailed as the child develops, and they can be called upon when needed.

There is a very important relationship between children's ability to differentiate from their objects and the presence or absence of internalized good-object memories. That is, the process of differentiation is dependent upon the prior introjection of supportive memories of the parents. Those children that have a sufficient supply of supportive memories of their parents are able to separate both physically and emotionally from them. Conversely, those children that are undersupplied with these memories are unable to do so. The

well-supported and emotionally filled child has memories (ultimately thousands of memories) of the loving parent to "fuel" her on
the adventure of life. To put it concretely, *the positive memories of
the mother*, which are gathered together in the child's inner world,
serve as a substitute for *the actual physical presence of the mother*.
Therefore, the well-cared-for child carries her mother internally
wherever she goes. Conversely, those unfortunate children who
have not received enough love, comfort, and support are not able to
build up enough positive memories of their parents to allow them to
separate. They will either physically remain with their parents, long
after healthy children have left, or cling to "new" individuals, whom
they symbolize as parents. The example of Cathy, who felt harassed
by her mother but would then panic if she did not get a call from her
every two hours, illustrates the relationship between the lack of
internalized good objects and the inability to differentiate.

As part of her research on differentiation, Mahler and her associates (1975) observed the importance of (assumed) internalized good
objects on the child's ability to separate and explore the world independently. They found that mothers who consistently responded to
their infants' needs in an appropriate manner had children who were
able to get further away from them (as measured by physical distance) when compared to the children of mothers who ignored or
misidentified those needs.

The existence of early memories of support can be demonstrated
under conditions of extreme distress. Healthy adults can occasionally get a brief glimpse of their unconscious good-object memories.
A dramatic example of this was described by Greenson (1978), who
as a young psychiatrist during World War II worked as the chief of
the combat fatigue section in an air force hospital. He was charged
with the care of a young aerial photographer who had been taking
photographs when his warplane was hit by antiaircraft fire; this rup-
tured a three hundred gallon fuel tank, which washed over him
(luckily not igniting) and trapped him in the bomb bay, where he
nearly drowned. The plane returned to base, and he was hospitalized
with severe ulcerations from the gasoline. During his recovery this
airman complained to a nurse that he was hearing words in his head
that he could not understand. Careful exploration by Greenson
revealed that the words he was hearing were *amosnell* and
domosnell, words that meant nothing to him consciously.

Greenson's examination of the airman's history revealed that he had been raised on a sheep ranch in Idaho and that his mother had died before his second birthday. Greenson asked him to write his father and ask if his mother had been born in Europe, because the air force intelligence officer who looked at the words thought them possibly to be of European origin. His father replied that his mother had been born in Belgium, and the intelligence officer simultaneously reported to Greenson that the words came from a Flemish lullaby and meant, "I must hurry, you must hurry."

This case demonstrates the existence of good objects in the unconscious of adults who were well cared for as children. The airman retrieved from his unconscious deeply comforting memories from his earliest interactions with his mother. These memories were called upon to calm him during the moment of his greatest anxiety. Thus one of the clearest overt signs in a child (or an adult for that matter) that he was supported early on in development is a sense of calm when stressed. People call upon their internalized good objects to support them all the time, although they may not be conscious of this process.

The parent's or caregiver's techniques for soothing and calming the distressed child forms part of the internalized good object, and these techniques are remembered and applied later in life. Conversely, those children that are reared in unsupportive or hostile environments miss out on the experience of being comforted as children and never learn to comfort themselves later in adulthood. As a hypothetical example, let us look at a seven-year-old boy who gets into his first fight and returns home crying with a magnificent bloody nose. First, let us assume that he returns to a "good enough mother" and guess at her response to this crisis. Upon seeing her son she would probably calm him by reassuring him that he will not be punished for fighting nor die from a bloody nose. She might then take him into the kitchen, lean his head back, explain to him that he should breathe through his mouth, and calmly wipe the terrifying blood away. Her calm demeanor and her sureness serve to reduce her son's panic and fears. Later in life if he is physically injured or psychologically distressed he will be able to recall memories of similar incidents from his past and calm himself without the presence of his mother.

Now let us turn to an unsupportive family and introduce the same little seven-year-old tyro with a bloody nose. Any number of psychologically damaging scenarios are possible to imagine. One mother might forbid the child to enter the house because his blood might stain the rug, another might shake the child angrily and demand that he go back and beat up the child who had bloodied his nose. A mother with a more primitive psychological development might become enraged and attempt to retaliate against the child who attacked her son, thus creating more rage and confusion in the already terrified son. One former patient came home with this type of injury, and her mother screamed and fled in horror out the back door. The little girl had to chase after her mother in a futile effort to get help. When poorly supported children grow into physical adulthood, they will be unable to comfort themselves when stressed, and demand instead that others take care of them. As we will see, a lack of positive memories plays a large role in the dynamics of both the batterer and his victim.

The Lack of Positive Introjects and the Fear of Abandonment

The formal term for lack of internalized positive memories of the parent is *introjective insufficiency,* and it has been cited as a key to understanding the borderline personality disorder by Gerald Adler (1985), a current object relations theorist. Fairbairn recognized early on that parents who consistently failed to emotionally support their children left them feeling so empty and vulnerable that they were unable to differentiate from their still-needed parents. His abused children in the Edinburgh foundling home had few if any memories of support or comfort of their dysfunctional parents, and, therefore, had no internal supplies to support them when they were separated. Like the motorist who is running out of gas, these children had to stick very close to their fuel supply.

The child with too few positive introjects cannot stand the stress of normal, developmentally appropriate separations during childhood. During development all of the deprived child's energy is focused on the parent, waiting for the needed affection and support that never comes. In adulthood the previously deprived individual is likely to throw herself at nearly anyone regardless of the suitability of that person as a partner because the fear of abandonment is so great. Her powerful need to seek out others to stay with (in order to banish the feeling of emptiness and aloneness) *overshadows all other considerations*, and her choice of partners often proves to be destructive. These bad choices are partially determined by a lack of internal memories of the good, comfort-giving parent, as the following case illustrates:

Julie came for her first appointment in a vague, almost dazed state. She described a life of apparent aimless drifting from place to place with no underlying life plan. She was a striking looking woman, over six feet tall, and quite beautiful. She was currently living with a man in a cabin deep in the woods of Vermont without running water or other amenities that one would expect. Her descriptions of her companion were so vague and changeable that I could not form any clear picture of him, but it appeared that he was abusive and taking advantage of her financially, sexually, and emotionally. She described a childhood of almost total rejection by her mother, who would not deign to touch her physically. She was cared for by her father and grandmother, who were psychologically at war with her mother. It was decided that she belonged on the father-grandmother side of the family, and she often stayed at her grandmother's house, which was located on the same property. As a young woman, she caught the attention of a booking agent who sent "girls" out to auto, electronic, and houseware shows. Julie's job was to stand on a rotating stage, dressed in a revealing sequined gown, touting the virtues of new lines of automotive or electronic products. She reported that she felt more warmth from the men who looked at her at these shows than she ever sensed in her family. Rather than staying alone during these out-of-town jobs, she would temporarily move in with the first man who offered to take her home. Her interest in sexuality was minimal to nonexistent; all that she was interested in was the physical presence of another person. Naturally, her vulnerability led to many abuses, which she saw as payment for the sense of "security" she derived from the presence of a person. She once went home with a woman, and derived the same sense of comfort from her presence as she did from that of a man. Her only demand of these seducers was that they hold her until she fell asleep. Her current relationship derived from her visit to New England, where she enrolled in a nontraditional college. She moved in with her new lover within a week of arriving for classes.

In effect Julie, and thousands of similarly emotionally undernourished people, experience life from the perspective of a frightened, lonely child. The lack of internalized memories of a comfort-giving parent, which was extreme due to her mother's active rejection of her, is a clear example of introjective insufficiency.

Among individuals of equal intelligence who have differing levels of introjects there is an enormous contrast in what they can accomplish in life. Those individuals with abundant internalized good objects can express their native talents and freely interact with others in a well-differentiated (separated) manner. Those with poor or minimal good introjects cannot let their natural talents flower, for they are forced by their needs to expend all their energy pursuing mothering, whether from their original parents or from "new" individuals whom they symbolize as parents. These adults cannot deal with the tasks of adulthood because they are preoccupied with their still living parents' every opinion, and they cannot separate enough to get on with their own lives. As mentioned previously, Fairbairn recognized that the undersupported child could not go forward, for to do so would close the door on all hope of future parenting from her objects.

Introjective Insufficiency in Novels

If we turn to Philip Roth's previously mentioned novel, *Portnoy's Complaint*, we can see that introjective insuffiency and lack of differentiation play a major role in the relationship between Alexander Portnoy and his mother. He is enslaved and controlled by his mother's rejection of him. No matter what his achievements in life, they are not enough to win the needed support from his mother. The novel demonstrates that Portnoy is unable to differentiate from his mother, and is forever engaged in an internal dialogue with her. He symbolically rather than physically returns to her, argues with her, begs for understanding from her, or just rails at the fact that she always rejects his best efforts. Portnoy also understands, from the very beginning, that it is impossible to reject his mother, even though she unfairly rejected him:

> When I am bad I am locked out of the apartment. I stand at the door hammering and hammering until I swear I will turn over a new leaf. But what is it I have done? I shine my shoes every

evening on a sheet of last night's newspaper laid carefully over linoleum; afterward I never fail to turn securely the lid on the tin of polish, and to return the equipment to where it belongs. I roll the toothpaste tube from the bottom, I brush my teeth in circles and never up and down, I say "Thank you" I say, "You're welcome," I say, "I beg your pardon," and "May I . . . " . . . Nonetheless, there is a year or so in my life when not a month goes by that I am told to pack my bag and leave. . . . Who cares! And out the door I go, into the long dim hallway. Who cares! I will sell newspapers on the streets in my bare feet . . . —and then it is enough for me to see the empty milk bottles standing by our welcome mat, for the immensity of all I have lost to come breaking over my head. (13–15)

This clever fictional mother has recognized that the more she rejects her son, the more power and control she will have over him. Portnoy is caught in what is technically called an "unresolved dependency." An unresolved dependency is an emotional Catch-22 in which the individual cannot separate until she feels fulfilled by her parent, and the parent, for whatever reason, cannot or will not cooperate. The reader may question the irrational aspect of this behavior and wonder why the adult with an unresolved dependency cannot choose another mothering object. The first obstacle to choosing a new "parent" is that the "adult" is really acting like one of Fairbairn's infants—she is *intensely* focused on the mother and no one else. Second, the abused or neglected child is enormously attached to the parent, out of guilt, as the child can see how pathetic the parent really is. Very often the child feels responsible for the parent's welfare, and could never bear to abandon the infantile parent.

Tragically, when deprived introjectively empty people do seek out new objects, they most often find new objects that bear a striking resemblance to their original rejecting objects. These are the "abusive partners" that are featured in the self-help literature. Once the rejecting object is imprinted on the child, she will seek out this style of relationship in the future. This tendency to find the very same frustrations in adulthood as one experienced in childhood is called *repetition compulsion,* and it will be discussed in chapter 5.

Portnoy's mother seems to possess the love and support that he so desperately requires. However, this is an illusion. That is, this mother *claims* that she is a self-sacrificing mother, and in fact she does perform some appropriate mothering tasks. However, on balance, she inhibits and rejects her son to a far greater extent than she supports him. What is more, she rejects organic aspects of her son, so that he becomes deeply ashamed of himself. The novel focuses on Portnoy's obsession with, and shame about, his sexuality, an organic aspect of him that is totally rejected by his mother. In reality, mothers and fathers like Sophie Portnoy are so involved with their own needs that they are unable to nurture the next generation. In effect, they sacrifice their own children's development in an attempt to satisfy their own unmet needs, unmet needs that are a consequence of the failures of the prior generation of parents.

Integration: The Third Development Process

The third fundamental developmental process that occurs as the ego matures is integration. This process occurs after differentiation has been established, since it requires that the individual realize that people are separate from him before he can merge their good aspects and bad aspects into a single view.

Like differentiation, integration has two meanings: one when applied to persons outside the self and one that applies to the self. First, when integration is used to describe the child's view of external objects, it refers to the recognition that a person outside the self can be frustrating at one moment, gratifying the next, and yet remain the same person. This is actually a major developmental achievement, because the child's young ego first experiences the gratifying mother as a separate person from the ungratifying mother. These part-object perceptions of the mother are referred to as the bad part-object representation and the good part-object representation.

Second, when *integration* is used about the self it refers to the individual's ability to acknowledge and experience the connectedness of separate feelings, moods, and behaviors. For instance, a well-integrated minister, priest, or rabbi will be able to accept his or her appropriate hostility despite the fact that in the role of religious leader she or he is directed to behave in a helpful, understanding, and altruistic manner. Later in this section I will present an extreme example of lack of integration of the self in an adult patient.

Integration of External Objects: Merging the "Separate Mothers" Into a Single Object

Early on the infant knows his mother only by the quality of the immediate interaction that occurs between them. Hamilton (1988) observed this lack of integration in a normal two-year-old-boy. Every morning when he was left at the baby-sitter's he would cry, protest, and shrink from the baby-sitter as if she were a rejecting object. He saw the baby-sitter as "bad," because she signaled the loss of his "good object" mother. As soon as the mother disappeared and the baby-sitter affectionately picked him up and hugged him, he would play happily with the other children. The sitter had shifted in his perceptions from a rejecting object to a gratifying object because of the affection that she provided him. When his mother returned in the afternoon the boy experienced his (abandoning) mother as a rejecting object and would ignore her presence, and say, "Bad Ma." His mother was remembered in two ways: as an abandoner and as a signal that he would now lose his good object baby sitter. After his mother would pick him up and hug him, he would switch his perception of her back to "good mother" and happily go home. The young child's inability to integrate the two experiences (abandonment and gratification) as separate parts of the same mother is at this age entirely normal. The child's inner world is not yet organized to the point that he can understand that the very same person can be gratifying at one moment and frustrating at a later one.

The process of integration gradually takes place in the developing child's inner world, beginning between the ages of three and four. The thousands upon thousands of gratifying events that occur over time slowly form predictable and coherent memories of the mother; the package of those rewarding memories with the mother form a positive inner picture of her. As we all know, a little rain has to fall in every infant's life, and there are going to be many occasions when the infant is "ungratified": irritated, inconsolable, or frustrated, simply because the mother is absent when the child needs her. These negative events, and the object associated with them, coalesce over time into an inner picture of the mother as bad or ungratifying. Technically, this inner image of the mother is called the *internalized rejecting object*. Those children who are reared in supportive environments have far fewer memories to compose the image of the

rejecting object, which is much weaker than the internalized gratifying object.

Over the first four years of childhood the well-cared-for child
begins to connect the two separate packages of memories together,
even though they have different emotional contents. This is possible
because the small package of negative memories of the mother,
resulting from the few times when she behaved in a frustrating manner, is not terribly frightening to the child. This is particularly true
when that package of memories is compared to the much larger body
of gratifying memories. The inner, previously separate, dual images
of the mother—the bad-ungratifying mother and the good-gratifying
mother—become a single, unified perception. This process has been
briefly noted before in the description of Mahler's final stage of individuation. This process is nonthreatening to the well-cared-for child
because the mother *is* almost completely "good"—there are very
few memories of frustration (and none of abuse) to fear. That is,
there are not enough frightening memories of the bad mother (now
recognized to be part of one mother) to upset the child. The number
of frustrating memories must be far fewer than the number of gratifying memories for integration to take place successfully. This is
because the merger of the two separate views of the mother will
expose the negative memories to the child's view. That is, the negative memories are no longer hidden in the separate mothering person previously categorized as the rejecting mother. The child's
increasingly structured ego can now tolerate a less-than-perfect
mother, or, to put it more accurately, a mother who puts certain limits on the child's behavior.

If, on the other hand, the rejecting, frustrating memories far out-
number the number of gratifying memories, then integration will not
occur, as the reality of the rejecting mother is too much for the young
child's psyche to bear. Technically, the achievement of the merger of
the two part-object views of the mother into a single whole-object
view is called *integration of part-object representations.*

Integration heralds the onset of healthy, mature ambivalence.
The child with a single view of his mother can experience opposite
feelings (though the negative feelings should be less powerful than
the positive ones) toward the same mother. Before integration the
child was free to kick and bite the rejecting part-object mother
because she was perceived as a completely different person from the

good mother. Now, with the achievement of integration, the four-year-old whose mother will not allow him to grab a candy bar at the check-out counter cannot easily fly into a rage at her because he remembers that this frustrating aspect is a very small part of his larger, gratifying mother. All of a sudden the child recognizes that he is risking a great deal in acting on his desire for a candy bar. The child's frustration of his immediate need is suddenly confronted by the totality of all the mother's "goodness": the four thousand feedings, the constant toileting, nose wipings, comforting, caregiving interactions that are available in his memory. The importance of a minor immediate gratification fades into obscurity when compared to the mass of remembered comforting interactions with his mother. The clash within the child between his angry desire for the candy bar and his new ability to remember his mother's "goodness" results in a considerable calming of his angry feelings. He is not as angry now because he can remember the overwhelming number of loving interactions that more than balance his current frustration. This dampening process is called, somewhat inappropriately, *neutralization of drives.*

The alert reader will wonder why the concept of drives suddenly reappears, since Fairbairn's position was that there was no such thing as free-floating drives. As I have noted previously, Freud assumed that humankind is motivated by instincts, and that beneath the civility and good will of well-adjusted humans there remained a cauldron of "toned down" drives. Fairbairn was at the extreme opposite end of the theoretical spectrum, in that he saw human beings as fundamentally good, and not struggling to suppress their antisocial, primitive instincts. He recognized that anger was a result of frustration of the child's legitimate developmental needs, and that attentive, loving mothers produce children with very little aggression. Fairbairn understood that the absence of aggression in these well-reared children was not the consequence of sublimation of intense instincts but rather the result of good parenting that *never produced much rage in the child in the first place.* He also recognized that you could create a monstrous, enraged human by depriving him at every opportunity. The fact that the deprived and frustrated child ends up as a dangerous, violent adult in no way proves that aggression is a basic component of the normal human personality.

The child blessed with good parents can calm down her internal demands because her ego structure is heavily populated by memories of abundant gratification in the past. This child can postpone her need for immediate gratification by consulting her memories of past gratifications. These memories allow her to "hold on" for a few more minutes because she is sure that some form of reward will be forthcoming, or, should the reward fail to appear, she will not be devastated because she has the comfort of past support. As the child matures she can do with less and less "tangible" gratifications, simply because she is supported by greater numbers of remembered comfort-giving interactions.

The Failure of Integration in Neglected and Abused Children

Integration cannot take place in the inner world of the neglected or deprived child. The reasons have already been alluded to a number of times in the section above. Integration allows the child to "see" both the loving-comforting and the frustrating-depriving parts of his mother as belonging to the same person. If the neglected-abused child somehow (it never happens in reality) forced herself to integrate the overwhelming number of nasty, thoughtless, hurtful interactions she has experienced with her mother with the very few positive memories of love and comfort, she would see that her mother is far more hateful and abusive than she is loving. *This is a perception that no child can tolerate.* The child must keep these perceptions separate and continue to see her mother (or father) as two different, unrelated persons. This is called *splitting,* and I have reserved chapter 4 for a thorough discussion of this critically important defense.

The frustrated, emotionally deprived child has a much greater problem controlling his real or imagined needs. The enormous pressure from previously unmet needs is the source of problems with self-control that are at the heart of so many personality disorders. The well-nurtured child in the earlier example who wanted the candy bar was not willing to risk either the loss of future rewards or the loss of his mother's good will for a moment of indulgence. He was able to delay gratification because he had access to an inner storehouse of memories of prior satisfactions as well as a realistic hope of future gratification. Using the same principle the rejected, empty child, with a meager and unreliable history of gratification with his mother, has no such storehouse of comforting memories to tap into and little hope for the future. This child will lose sight of the goodness in his mother (which was never strongly established in the first place) when he is deprived of the candy. All his need will be focused on the candy, and his mother will appear to be blocking an important source of gratification. This unintegrated perception of his mother can easily lead to a mother/child brawl. Aggression toward his mother is a real possibility, because the child sees her under these conditions as totally frustrating. In his perceptions the frustrating part of her is lodged in a completely separate person from the gratifying parts of her. This is exactly the opposite internal situation from that of the child with an available and gratifying mother who was inhibited from acting out his desire by his memories of past satisfactions. Thus, the rage of the deprived child is not inhibited by pressure from memories of love. The child's rage is based on his inability to tolerate frustration of any type, since he is always internally frustrated. Satisfaction of *any type* appears to be enormously important to the developmentally deprived child. The intense desire for nonhuman satisfaction was termed "substitute satisfactions" by Fairbairn, who saw addiction, alcoholism, and other attempts to fill up the empty self as a consequence of a loss of hope for human closeness. Note the difference between the expression of drives in Fairbairn's model in comparison with Freud's. Freud saw the expression of intense needs as the building blocks of personality while Fairbairn saw them as the consequence of the breakdown of human relating.

Parents who have failed to nurture their children early in the child's development (the first five years of life) almost universally report that, as the child grows older, he becomes increasingly willful and unmanageable. It is easy for the dysfunctional mother (or father) to push aside the needs of an infant, but the empty teen-aged child, who is pressured by fourteen years of unmet needs and filled with rage at being emotionally or physically abandoned, is a far more difficult person to ignore:

> When separation anxiety is seen in this light, as a basic human disposition, it is only a small step to understand why it is that threats to abandon a child, often used as a means of control, are so very terrifying. . . . Not only do threats of abandonment create intense anx-

iety but they also arouse anger, often also of intense degree, especially in older children and adolescents. This anger, the function of which is to dissuade the attachment figure from carrying out the threat, can easily become dysfunctional. It is in this light, I believe, that we can understand such absurdly paradoxical behavior as the adolescent, reported by Burnham (1965), who, having murdered his mother, exclaimed, "I couldn't stand to have her leave me."　(Bowlby 1988:30–31)

As we will discover during the discussion of the battering scenario, physical assaults upon the very person upon whom the deprived child-adult is insecurely attached are commonplace. It is the male child who, when severely deprived, has a good chance of becoming a needy, short-tempered, batterer of women, while the deprived female child has an equally good chance of growing up to be the victim of battering.

Integration of the "Self"

As mentioned previously, integration refers both to merging of the two external part-object views of people outside the self as well as to an internal integration of the various parts of the self. At the same time that the child sees the mother as two separate objects (gratifying and frustrating), she sees herself as two different persons as well. When the parent behaves in a loving, responsive and gratifying manner, the child perceives herself as "good"—i.e., loved, important, and cared for. Conversely, when the mother frustrates the child's needs, the child experiences herself as "bad"—i.e., worthless, hated, and unimportant. Integration of the self occurs when the child is able to see herself as the same person regardless of the responses of the parent. This important developmental achievement is called self-constancy, and it cannot occur until the child has achieved object constancy. The child with self-constancy will feel secure even when her mother is temporarily angry at her.

There is more to integration of the self than the simple merger of the good and bad selves into a single self. There are subtle aspects of the self that have to be acknowledged as being parts of the whole personality—parts that may have been disapproved of by the parents. The previous example of Alexander Portnoy from Philip Roth's novel is illustrative of the difficulty of integrating sexuality into the self when the overpoweringly important mother has repeatedly rejected that part of the child. A well-integrated self has the ability to see and accept all parts of the self as connected and operating as a single unit. During childhood controlling parents force their children to conceal parts of themselves that the parents cannot tolerate. Another common aspect of the child's self that is rejected is anger, and many children are "told" that they are not angry when they indeed are. In other, more severe, cases the child might be punished so severely for his display of anger that he represses all awareness of it completely. The most extreme example of lack of integration within the self that I have found comes from a case report on a patient suffering from an almost total collapse of his ego structure. Like Freda and Greta, the undifferentiated twins, extreme examples of psychopathology make the point about these human ego process most clearly. The following example is not representative of the lack of integration in character disorders, for it is more severe; however, it does illustrate one person's experience of this extreme state:

> He no longer knew which parts of his parents he was made of, and each piece had a nationality: his father was English, his mother German/Polish, who now lives in England. Each "piece" had a special and separate characteristic. His father is a professor, but in addition was a military man through family tradition, but at the same time a pacifist; he is upper and lower class, conservative and socialist, etc. He began to believe that his mother was Jewish. He gave a nationality to each of these "pieces": one "piece" of him was Prussian , and very rigid, one "piece" English, one "piece" Polish, etc. Then he wanted to become a Jew and soon after he no longer wanted to. First he admired them, then he criticized them.
> (Rey 1979:458)

This example illustrates the inner experience of an individual who is unable to integrate all the parts that went into the development of his sense of self. The lack of coherence within the ego structure leads to an inability to tie all the disparate parts of the personality together. A poorly integrated ego leaves the unfortunate person on the brink of chaos. This is yet another "key" reason (there seem to be about a dozen "key" reasons that contribute to adult personality disorders) that the poorly reared child develops into an adult who is confused, chaotic, and easily taken over by others. The poorly integrated individual has so many contradictory views of himself, and of others, that he loses all confidence in his perceptions, feelings, and opinions. He is easy prey for people who (to him forcefully) present another version of reality, for he is so unsure of his own shifting and chaotic view. Lack of integration plays an important role in any situation where a clash of opinions occurs. This is particularly true in the battering scenario, where the dominant individual forces the submissive partner to accept his distorted view of reality.

Summary

The most important concepts in the development of the child's personality are the three fundamental ego development processes that must be completed for a healthy personality to emerge. The first process that the child must master is the awareness of differentiation, in terms of both inner and outer reality. First, she must learn that she is a separate person from her external objects, and she must learn the differences between shades of her own inner experience. In terms of differentiation from objects the developing child has to learn to experience herself as a separate and independent person in the world. Those children who are poorly nurtured by their parents remain undifferentiated because 1. they cannot separate from their neglectful parent for fear of losing out on the love and support that they still need, and 2. as adults they remain undifferentiated because they receive comfort from feeling the presence of their depriving objects "inside" themselves. The second aspect of healthy differentiation relates to the individual's ability to experience subtle difference of feelings from other relatively similar feelings in their inner world. The child is helped in this task by the good enough mother who has accurate perceptions of his needs, and helps him to learn to recognize and label his inner feelings correctly. Conversely, the poorly reared child does not have accurate responses to his needs, and is not able to identify one need or feeling state from another.

The second process that occurs simultaneously with differentiation is introjection. Introjection is the process whereby the child takes in events and interactions with the mother and categorizes them into clusters of similar memories. Clusters of nurturing events in which the child was loved and supported by the mother become the internalized good object, while clusters of memories in which the child was frustrated and rejected by his mother become the internalized rejecting object. Positive, supportive memories are continuously called upon during stress to stabilize the ego and impart a sense of calm to the child. Negative memories have the opposite effect in that they undermine the child's sense of worth and make her more susceptible to stress. When the child lives in a neglectful or abusive world, she will have few positive internalized memories of her objects and will be unable to face the normal stresses of life. Moreover, the unfortunate child (and, later, adult) who has such an abundance of negative memories of her objects not only feels undersupported and easily panicked but also must engage in defensive techniques to keep from remembering the parental abuses.

The last process that the ego must accomplish for a healthy personality to emerge is integration, which, like differentiation, has one meaning when applied to external objects and another when applied to the self. In terms of external objects, the child must integrate his early perception that his mother is actually two separate people, one good and the other bad, into a single view. The achievement of this important form of integration requires that the child's positive memories of interactions with his parents must far outweigh the memories of negative or frustrating interactions. If the reverse is true, with frustrating memories outweighing the gratifying memories, then integration will not take place. Integration of the gratifying and rejecting parts of the parents "exposes" the rejecting parts as belonging to the mother (or father), whereas previously they had been split off into a separate person (the rejecting parent). No child can tolerate the constant awareness that he is hated or continually rejected by his intensely needed parents. If the neglected child does manage to integrate the large package of negative memories with the smaller package of positive memories, he will be faced with a reality that will make him overwhelmingly anxious. His solution is to keep the two packages of memories apart in his inner world. Integration also refers to the individual's ability to experience himself as a single coherent unity. It requires that the child acknowledge all parts of himself, which allows his ego to meld all the different part-selves into one coherent and functional sense of self.

The reader can see that when the child has nurturing parents development is positive, but when things go wrong the unmet needs and ego deficiencies unite to create a major personality disorder. Let us look at the worst-case scenario. The child who is so unfortunate as to be born to a depressed, alcoholic, single mother will receive so little early support that he will not be able to develop enough positive internalized memories to allow him to leave his inadequate mother for an instant. He will never develop a sense of separateness from her because differentiation feels like abandonment. That is, he has no internal "fuel" to sustain himself apart from her. Similarly, he will remain unintegrated because negative memories of neglect by his mother far outweigh positive memories of support from her. His anger and rage will increase over time because of the constant frustration of his legitimate needs, and these frustrations will not be tempered by larger memories of his mother's love and acceptance. Thus we end up with an "adult" who is enormously dependent, who collapses under the slightest of stresses, who cannot tolerate the smallest frustration, who—because he is unintegrated—sees others in black-and-white ways, and who has to hide from his emptiness and pain through substitute satisfactions (perhaps alcohol or drugs). This is the psychological portrait of the future batterer.

CHAPTER THREE

Personality Disorders:
The View from
the Outside

he concept of personality disorders was already introduced in
chapters 1 and 2. This chapter continues that discussion of a
diverse group of disorders by focusing on observable behavior typical of these individuals. These are the men who become batterers
and the women who become their victims. Battering does not occur
in a vacuum, but rather takes place when people with specific psychological characteristics, not all of which directly relate to battering itself, join together in a relationship. Not all individuals with
character disorders end up as batterers or victims, since this diagnostic group is so large and diverse; however, nearly all adult batterers and adult victims of repeated abuse come from this group.

Interestingly, this diagnostic group has been known since Freud's
time, and their overt characteristics were well recognized by the
therapeutic community of that era. However, they were not dealt
with frequently in the early years of psychoanalysis because they
could not tolerate the discipline and compliance required for psychoanalytic treatment, and because they were unable to develop
and maintain consistent transferences to the analyst. After all, what
self-respecting character disorder—likely to be alcoholic, short-
tempered, impulsive, grandiose, and excessively aggressive—would
tolerate lying down on the couch three times a week? Because of
these individuals' defiance of the strict demands of classical psychoanalysis, they were thought to be completely "un-analyzable."
This was true at that time: one either conformed to the demands of

the treatment or went without; there were no alternatives available. Today there are many different forms of psychotherapy that do not make the rigid demands of classical psychoanalysis, and these newer therapies have allowed many character disordered individuals to receive treatment. This chapter focuses on overt behaviors that express the underlying structural problems discussed in chapter 2. The reader now knows that the ego structures of these individuals are underdeveloped in three areas: 1. the inability to successfully differentiate their sense of self from others, 2. the introjection of too few positive early memories to support their sense of self in times of stress, and 3. the inability to integrate the positive and negative images of their objects into a single whole object. Each of the characteristics described in this chapter is common in both the male batterer and his female victim, and they are presented to give the reader a full perspective of the psychological reality in which these individuals live.

Personality Disorders: The Independent and Dependent Patterns

Before I launch into the specific characteristics of character disorders it is important to mention the two general "styles" these disorders take. For the sake of simplicity I will call one style of the disorder the independent pattern and the other the dependent pattern. Keep in mind that there are many exceptions to this general rule, but I estimate that 70 percent of male character disorders use the independent pattern and, similarly, 70 percent of female character disorders use the dependent pattern.

Surprisingly, adults with character disorders who use the independent pattern often appear to be nearly the *opposite* when compared to those individuals who use the dependent pattern, despite the fact that they are afflicted by the same basic disorder. Independents tend to exaggerate their sense of sureness about themselves, their sense of personal power, and, most importantly, their lack of need for others. The greatest contrast between the two patterns is the independents' ability to conceal all overt expressions of their enormous dependency needs. He or she appears to be able to live without others forever. Conversely, those individuals who use the dependent pattern appear to be psychologically starving to death when she or he is without a partner.

Men who use the independent pattern may live alone, engage in reckless, or at least exciting forms of behavior, and appear to be supremely desirable to many women. Many men who use the independent pattern (but not all) spend an inordinate amount of time and effort making themselves attractive through exercise and the purchase of expensive clothes or other self-indulgent items, including fashionable autos or expensive sports equipment. Despite their superficial desirability, when these men become involved with women they tend to act selfishly and tyrannically.

Some number of women also use the independent pattern. They too appear extremely desirable, and are often single; some enjoy athletics, while others focus all their energy on their jobs. Many independent-style women occupy powerful positions involving great responsibility. The example of June, a broadcasting executive, will be described below. Diagnostically, individuals that use the independent pattern are usually classified as narcissistic personality disorders, because their behavior is self-centered and arrogant. The narcissistic personality can be conceptualized as the independent version of the borderline personality disorder.

The dependent pattern or style appears to be nearly opposite the independent pattern. Women who use the dependent pattern seem to be lonely, desperate, and excessively dependent on others. When a man comes into their lives they may give up their own interests and adopt the interests of their new partner. In general the female partner who uses the dependent pattern will submerge her weak sense of self into the male partner's pseudo strength. This is also true of dependent pattern men, like John, the furniture maker who was described in the introduction. He abandoned his own preferences, profession, and interests, and adopted the world and lifestyle of his female partners.

Despite their overt need for a partner, women who use the dependent pattern often find it difficult to find a suitable mate. If, for instance, a dependent pattern female becomes involved with an untroubled man, problems are likely to emerge almost immediately. The dependent pattern personality disorder will live in fear that her "normal" partner will discover how weak and insecure she really feels. She will have to attempt to hide her unreliability, her inability to control her outbursts of temper, or other forms of acting out. Surprisingly, the chance for a "successful" relationship (if I may use that phrase when describing characterological relationships) will improve if she finds a male character disorder that uses the typical male pattern. This is due to the fact that her similarly disordered partner will accept her acting out, and she will not live in fear that her "real self" will be discovered.

Outward appearances are deceiving, and the two opposite appearing patterns have more in common than meets the eye. We will discover that the hyperindependent male is awash in unmet dependency needs from his childhood, which he constantly struggles to keep at bay. When a well-adjusted woman is unlucky enough to become involved with this type of man she will discover how tyrannical and demanding he can be. He will squeeze her dry in the process of getting his needs met, and will then discard her. The independent pattern of this disorder has greater control over the expression of unmet infantile needs; however, they are still present, and as powerful as the needs in both men and women who use the dependent pattern. Men, as opposed to women, who use the independent pattern differ on the dimension of aggression, in that they will force their partners to meet their needs. They often demand immediate gratification, and, as we will see in the battering syndrome, many will resort to physical violence when their partners cannot meet their unreasonable and insatiable demands.

Despite the fact that most character disordered men use the independent pattern, with most similarly disordered women staying within the dependent pattern, there are many exceptions, such as John, mentioned above, who became engulfed by his girlfriend's horse-boarding business. The following example of June shows the reverse, a woman who uses the independent pattern:

June was forced to come to therapy by her physician, who had treated her for a severe physical illness brought about by chronic overwork and exhaustion. June came to her first therapy session with three textbooks on abnormal psychology. Instead of describing her problems, she asked me a series of pointed questions designed to help her make her own diagnosis. Our session was repeatedly interrupted by calls from her beeper, and her greatest concern was to locate a phone in the building so that she could return the calls as soon as our session was over. June spoke hurriedly, as if her recent physical illness and her appearance in my office were minor irritants that were interfering with her busy agenda. She had started working immediately after high school at a local television station as the "weather girl." Her good looks, self-assurance, and unvarnished ambition soon helped her move into television reporting, and then into advertising sales. She watched the studio engineer, and her interest prompted him to help her learn the technical side of broadcasting, which led to her FCC license. Her capacity for work seemed unlimited, and she filled in for other staff members who were either absent or on vacation, often learning their jobs in a surprisingly short time. As it turned out, June's capacity for work was equivalent to her desire for power and control, and she ran her life like a one-person corporation. All activity was guided by the principle of more: more information, more success, more power, more money. She lived extremely frugally and gradually bought a larger and larger interest in the station until it was almost all hers. Her weekends were devoted to the pursuit of an undergraduate degree, which had been postponed by her rapid immersion into the business world, and to developing and directing television commercials for local businesses. Her interpersonal world was frantic and nearly all her social contacts were based on business. She reported that she was currently living with a man who was lazy and often resisted her demands. Interestingly, she also reported that many of her employees also appeared to resist the demands that she placed upon them, but she was unaware that her uncompromising nature was the source of passive resentment from others. From her description, she had already experienced several similar relationships with men who were not up to her "speed." June never felt abandoned (though she felt lonely), for her feelings of abandonment were banished by her frenetic lifestyle. The only visible source of anxiety in her life were those situations in which she felt exploited and demeaned, or felt unable to exert direct control. For instance, she once entered a meeting with three potential advertisers and was initially mistaken for the television station's secretary. This infuriated her internally, and she became extremely dominating in the meeting, thus leaving no doubt in the minds of others as to her power and status. June's family history was fraught with role reversals, in that she acted as the adult to her incompetent and chaotic parents, and virtually raised her younger siblings as well. Her mother exploited her organizational and intellectual skills unmercifully, and June felt responsible for the well-being of the entire family. She had to negotiate with welfare agencies, the police, and the many merchants to whom her parents owed money. She even had to learn to read maps at a young age because her parents would repeatedly get lost while driving. Despite her best efforts, June was unable to influence the direction that her family was taking, and she had the endless task of coping with the mistakes that her parents continued to make. Even though her judgments and efforts often saved the family from disaster, she was never given credit. In fact, her mother constantly blamed her for everything that went wrong. As a consequence June learned to be alert at all times for any hint of criticism, and developed the skills of a professional debater to deflect her mother's verbal attacks. As an adult these skills aided her in business; she could not be intimidated and would argue her positions relentlessly. Her childhood was suffused with chronic anxiety, since she felt continually overburdened with responsibility—almost as if the world would stop if she relaxed for a moment. This resulted in a chronic, angry, defensive approach to others, which alienated her staff, who in her view never worked hard enough. She had a peculiar double standard where her autonomy was concerned. For instance, if an executive of the network with which her station was affiliated asked her to make a business trip, no matter how inconvenient for her, she would always do so willingly. The epitome of this occurred when she was on vacation in Maine with her boyfriend and was asked to fly to Washington for a meeting. She did so without hesitation, and berated her boyfriend for complaining about her behavior. However, if any demand was placed upon her by persons not important to her success, she would experience even greater feelings of being overwhelmed, and she used this feeling to justify ignoring those demands completely.

When we compare June to John, we can see that women who use the independent style tend to attract male character disorders who use the dependent style. Not surprisingly, June clashed with character disordered men who used the independent style: she would become competitive in regard to their power, professional status, or relative importance. Male character disorders cannot tolerate direct competition from a woman who uses the same style; in fact, they are repelled by women like June. On the other hand, passive and dependent men were very attracted to her, for they could have their unrecognized dependency needs satisfied. In return they had to give up all vestiges of initiative. Very often, they became covertly rebellious and passive-aggressive. Interestingly, our culture tends to see females who use the independent pattern, like June, as abnormal, while males who have the very same type of psychopathology are admired and celebrated as tough go-getters. In either case, male or female, the personality disorder who uses the independent pattern is simply living out the end result of a childhood that distorted the development of his or her sense of self.

I would like to add yet another level of complexity in regard to alternation within the same person of the two patterns. I have been witness to a number of situations where the independent/dependent roles of the partners reversed over time. That is, the partner who originally used the independent pattern reversed and switched to the dependent pattern, and vice versa:

Carl was a country and western songwriter-singer who lived a life as superficially colorful as the characters in his ballads. He had spent most of his time on the road with his band. Travel, alcohol, and increasing difficulties with his third wife and his children from a previous marriage brought him reluctantly to my office. He described his childhood in East Texas as an endless (but unrecognized by him at the time) series of emotional frustrations. His father was a local politician and oil-well equipment dealer who raised him "by the book." The book was the Bible, and his father used it to keep Carl at emotional arm's length from him. His mother was a pathetic, bitter woman, who saw herself as a member of high society from the East Coast who had been "temporarily" exiled to Texas. She was a music teacher who wrote romantic songs, and lived under the delusion that her songs would make her famous back in New York and Philadelphia. Her maternal skills were minimal, and she dealt with Carl as if he were a continuously annoying, coarse intruder into her life of music and sophistication. Most of the child-raising chores were assigned to a hired woman who, Carl remembered, would often fall asleep while "caring" for him. He recalled begging to be let into his mother's music room when she was working, but being turned away. Carl was never physically disciplined, and suffered from neglect rather than abuse. Like many neglected children, Carl often felt vengeful and rebelled against both parents. He particularly despised his father's "sermons," since he experienced the lack of warmth between them. The hypocrisy of being identified as a son of this man, who was presenting himself to the world as a parent while taking his "parenting" instructions from a book, was too much for Carl to bear. As luck would have it, Carl inherited the talent that his mother had no opportunity to develop, and at a young age was playing musical instruments and composing songs, often (covertly hostile) parodies of her efforts. As a college student he rebelled as strongly as he could against his conventional, conservative upbringing, living a life antithetical to everything his parents believed in. Most conspicuously, he preyed on women, younger than himself, who were drawn to his musical talent and growing fame. He took particular pleasure in the pursuit, conquest, and then abandonment of one woman after another and felt on some level that he was getting back at his mother for her indifference toward him. His strategies for these conquests were conscious and played out with great finesse. He often went for the most vulnerable and dependent women, who were easily impressed with his talent. The moment he was sure of their attachment to him, he would abandon them in ways designed to maximize their pain. In adulthood he lived a seminomadic life with his band, but over the years he married several times and had two children who often traveled with him. He finally met a woman in whom he felt enough interest to marry without misgivings, because of his increased vulnerability to age and an unconscious recognition that his latest partner was somehow reminiscent of his mother. This woman tapped into his unacknowledged dependency needs. The moment they had settled down, his new wife became increasingly critical of his teen-aged children. Within two months she demanded that they leave and live with their hapless biological mother in Arizona. Carl felt unable to protect his children from his wife's demands, for his deeply repressed need for parenting took precedence over their interests. He became more and more servile after he sent his children away, and his wife increased her demands upon him until he was almost housebound. She would not allow him to socialize with his old band members, and kept him busy with trivial house chores while she worked as a secretary. He tested his wife's resolve by secretly spending a weekend with his old musician friends, and when she discovered his defection, she locked him out of their house and systematically destroyed his most prized musical instruments. He begged her for forgiveness, and as a condition of his return, his wife placed increased levels of constraint on him. Not surprisingly, Carl's use of alcohol increased dramatically, and he began to experience crying spells for which he had no explanation. The pattern had come full circle, with Carl now trapped at home and abandoned by his second desperately needed parental object.

This type of case history is not uncommon, and it should alert the reader to the underlying reality that men who were abandoned in childhood are not that different, in terms of their fundamental pathology, from abandoned women. The differences lie mainly in the ability of men (and women) who use the independent pattern to inhibit the overt expression of their powerful dependency needs. Carl was very successful at this strategy early in life; however, it broke down as he became older and his deeply buried needs for the parenting that he never received reappeared.

I have gone into some detail about the overt styles that individuals with personality disorders use because I want the battering relationship to be understood in the larger context of psychological dysfunction. Battering typically occurs when a man who uses the independent pattern becomes involved with a woman who uses the dependent pattern. I do not want to imply that the psychological similarities between the independent and dependent patterns excuse, or in anyway reduce, the tragic outcome that results from domestic violence. Despite the fact that these patterns are psychologically similar, the consequences of domestic violence are extremely *dissimilar* for the two groups. Men who turn into batterers inflict grievous, often fatal injuries on their spouses, while the reverse is rare. Once again I will turn to the Council of Scientific Affairs of the American Medical Association for an analysis of the violence done to women:

> In general, men perpetrate more aggressive actions against their female partners than women do against their male partners, and men perpetrate more severe actions and are more likely to perpetrate multiple aggressive actions against their partners during a single incident than are women against their male partners. In combination with men's greater average physical strength, these factors lead to quite different outcomes for women and men. Women are much more likely to be injured by their male partners than men are by their female partners. Over 80 percent of all assaults against spouses and ex-spouses result in injuries, com-

pared with 54 percent of the victims of stranger violence; victims of marital violence also have the highest rates of internal injuries and unconsciousness. (Browne 1992:3,186)

Thus, the battering scenario involves two individuals who are remarkably similar in terms of their inner psychology, but because they adopt different gender-based patterns of fulfilling their unmet needs, one group is physically abused and the other inflicts the abuse. Worse, the injustice of physical abuse has been, and still is, minimized by the legal system with only moderate punishment meted out to men who batter their partners.

A Reader's Guide to the Observable Characteristics of Personality (Character) Disorders

In this section I will illustrate the types of behaviors that can be seen in individuals who end up in battering relationships. As I have mentioned previously, I present the battering relationship as part of a larger dysfunctional system that involves many inappropriate behaviors in addition to the battering behavior itself.

The two diagnoses, *character disorders* and *personality disorders*, are used interchangeably. In general the individual must show a number of these characteristics over a long period of time to be diagnosed as a personality disorder. I have created four separate categories of behavior that are easily observable by the nonprofessional. They are 1. a low tolerance for frustration and impulsivity, 2. a lack of "deep" attachments to others, 3. extreme dependency on others, and, 4. a sense of personal shame and inadequacy, resulting in an inability to tell the truth and an avoidance of responsibility. The central issue of Fairbairn's "return to the bad object," which I introduced in the last chapter, and the complex reasons for its destructive power over people who are caught in its grip will be examined in great detail in chapter 5. Readers will find the seeds of the return to the bad object in each one of the four separate categories that are illustrated in this chapter.

Low Tolerance for Frustration and Impulsivity

In this first section I will look at impulsive, poorly planned, and self-defeating behaviors that are the result of the individual's underdeveloped ego. The poorly structured ego is not able to cope with tension that results from either external or internal sources. As we have seen, when the structure of the individual's ego is poor there will be few means for the control of tension. This is partially due to introjective insufficiency, which has been defined as a lack of enough comforting memories to support the person from the inside while combating pressure from the outside. If we return to the example of the airman who was nearly drowned in hot gasoline, we can see that his automatic reaction to this life-threatening catastrophe was to recall deeply unconscious memories of his comfort-giving mother. When disaster struck he was able to control his anxiety by tapping into the inner resources already accessible in his unconscious. The early memories became "structure" (complex pathways and resources that are activated when needed) in the matrix of his ego. The greater the structure, the more stress the individual can tolerate without experiencing the collapse of the ego's integrity. In terms of individuals involved in battering relationships, low tolerance for frustration is the key characteristic of the male batterer.

Acting Out The most direct and primitive way of dealing with inner tension that overwhelms the ego is to expel it by discharging it through acting out behaviors. *Acting out* is defined as the discharge, through action or speech, of tension the moment it is experienced. Tension must be discharged because the character disordered individual has no mechanisms to cope with it internally. The transformation of inner tensions into external activity solves many immediate problems for the personality disorder for it allows her to discharge the stress that she cannot handle, while simultaneously obscuring the original source of the tension. The penalty for acting out is that it produces greater problems for the person in the future. The activity, excitement, and tension discharge inherent in acting out blocks the specific emotionality (emptiness, boredom, abandonment) that originally motivated the behavior. As a consequence the individual who uses acting out to solve her immediate problems remains unsure of her motivations, and finds herself in one difficulty after another without any clear idea as to how she got there. Acting out is one of the most pathological consequences of inner emptiness and the lack of ego structure, as the following example illustrates:

Mary came into therapy because of her overuse of alcohol and the chaotic breakup of her most recent relationship. She was a psychiatric nurse who had much professional success but few friends outside work. She could not understand how her bitter and cynical attitude, her jealousy, demandingness, and attraction to men as disturbed as herself led to the chaos and physical abuse in her life. She had been in the area for only ten months, saying she had transferred to Vermont from a hospital in the same corporate chain because she thought New England was clean, pure, and filled with nice people. Her unrealistic idealization of this locale broke down within the year, and she began looking for yet another job site. All her chronic inner tension was dealt with by external acting out. For instance, she was the picture of physical health because of her program of daily jogging. Exploration revealed that the motivation for her exercise was to discharge unendurable tension. The ordinary stresses of her nursing job would build up in her to the point where she felt she had to either jog or explode. She described one extremely stressful day when she couldn't exercise because of a damaged tendon. She saw a young woman jogging down the road on her way home and was so filled with undifferentiated rage, envy, and tension that she had to pull off the road to vomit. Her relationships with men were fraught with jealousy and suspicion, and she invariably accused her (enormously unreliable) boyfriends of planning to "dump" her. She would often meet her boyfriends at her house after work for sex, which was another way that she relieved her inner tension. If her boyfriend of the moment failed to show up at the appointed time, she would become enraged and assume that she was either being abandoned or cheated on. These powerful feelings would cause her to drive around town, desperately looking for her boyfriend's car. Her search missions often resulted in bitter accusations and mutual physical assaults. In therapy we began to explore Mary's relationship with her overly seductive father, who used to take her out on "dates" when she was a teen-ager, leaving her mother home in an enraged and impotent state. Often her mother would then seek revenge on her daughter by bluntly rejecting her normal needs. Whenever I began to explore this material with her she would develop a severe headache and leave the session before the hour was up. She tried to maintain the illusion that she had "perfect parents" and that there was nothing wrong with her. Often after our sessions she would drink excessively to blunt the feelings of abandonment rising in her, calling her father once she was inebriated.

Acting out is one of the major techniques used by character disordered individuals to hide from the constant pain of feelings of abandonment. Mary was unlike typical battered women who get abused again and again by the same partner in that she was involved in a series of short-term, hostile, and extremely dependent relationships with four different men while she was seeing me. Two of these relationships involved physical violence between Mary and her partners. Her ego structure was very weak because she had so few positive internalized memories of her objects. Like many individuals with this type of disorder, she felt that the source of all her problems was "outside" herself, and she lived a nomadic life in response to tensions that constantly arose in her inner world. Acting out by moving from place to place was the only way that she could deal with her distress. The reader may ask why I didn't "talk some sense into her" by pointing out how empty her childhood was, how demanding and physically violent she herself was, and how her cherished father had used her for his own inappropriate vicarious sexual gratification. Don't forget that a person who has a history like Mary's has very little trust in *anyone*—including me. Moreover, she needed her rejecting parents (even though she was a chronological adult) perhaps ten times as much as a healthy person of her age because she was still waiting and longing for the nurturance that she lacked from her deprived childhood. Any negative comments about her desperately needed parents were met with defensive denial.

Violent Forms of Acting Out and the Role of Integration. The example of Mary brings us to the issue of violence in relationships. One of the most common forms of acting out in males who use the independent pattern is direct physical aggression. Fairbairn recognized that hate and aggressiveness in children were responses to frustration of their needs. Aggression is not an innate drive, as Freud originally claimed, but rather a consequence of extreme frustration. The deprived child is both enraged by his deprivation and yet needy and dependent, like the previously described fourteen-year-old inmate who had beaten and molested a number of younger children, but was still sucking his thumb. Frustration of the infant's needs provokes anger, which when translated into behavior appears as kicking, screaming, and general irritability. As mentioned previously, the unintegrated infant experiences two separate mothers. The mother or caregiver is experienced as completely and eternally "bad" when the infant is frustrated, because the child has no sense of the "good" mother while in this deprived state. The infant also assumes that the bad mother is a completely different person from the good mother. The mother does not even have to be present to be the bad mother, since frustration occurs when the child's needs are not met, whether the caregiver is present or not. In other cases the bad mother can be the actual mother who makes things worse for the child, perhaps by punishing the already deprived and enraged infant.

Over time severely deprived children grow up to be angry and dependent adults. This turns out to be a very volatile combination, for the "adult" with an entire childhood of unmet needs is in constant danger of exploding when he feels deprived. This explosiveness of the unintegrated adult exists because he still experiences his adult partner as "all bad" when he is frustrated, and therefore his attack on her seems to be justified. This extreme and unrealistically negative perception of the current partner is fueled by the thousands of memories of frustration from childhood, and these memories produce a rage-driven response. The individual acts as if he were attacking a mortal enemy rather than the wife who is temporarily frustrating him. As we will see, lack of integration, technically called *splitting* when it occurs in adulthood, is one of the ego problems that allow many male character disorders to become physically abusive.

The well-integrated person has the ability to experience outside individuals as integrated "whole objects." The process of integration, which was described as the child's dawning recognition that the frustrating mother and the gratifying mother are actually the same person, allows the healthy adult to experience the external frustrating object as a very small part of the whole "other." The following example of Sam illustrates how a critical lack of integration played a key role in the emergence of his physical violence toward his partners:

Sam was raised in a violent and dysfunctional household. His father, a small-town physician, was physically violent toward both his wife and Sam. His outbursts would often occur at the dinner table; he would lift Sam right out of his chair, take him into the living room, and beat him violently, often kicking him while he curled up for protection on the floor. His mother and younger brother would remain seated while these assaults took place. He reported that the most enraging and humiliating aspect of these beatings was his father's demand that he return to the table and finish his dinner as if nothing had happened. At other times his parents would leave him alone and go off with his younger, favored brother, and Sam would be left alone to his own devices. He remembered spending day after day fantasizing that he had a secret family in England who really loved and cherished him. Many of his fantasies revolved around their sudden arrival, and the announcement that they were reclaiming him as their lost son and taking him with them back to England. As a young adult Sam felt a great inertia and deadness inside him. He was attracted to women who had histories as poor as his own. Typically his relationships would begin with promise and excitement, but after a few months he would become increasingly sullen and silent and demand that his partner talk to him and carry the entire burden of relating. This became more and more difficult as his various partners found it impossible to remain cheery and pleasant when faced with a sullen, silent, demanding man. Eventually Sam would erupt in violence. During his violence toward his partners, Sam experienced them as all bad, which allowed him to feel justified in his rage.

Sam displayed the general pattern of males who abuse women. This potent combination of early deprivation and unintegrated perceptions will be examined in greater detail in chapters 4 and 5.

A telling aspect of the violence committed by character disorders is that it is most often directed at "innocent" others rather than the original parents. This is understandable in light of the neglected child's increased dependency on his parents (no matter what his or her age). Direct anger toward the parents is almost always inhibited because they are so necessary for the survival of the child or the now adult-child. The enraged child might torture animals or plug up school toilets, but he will never attack his parents directly. This does not mean that there is no conflict, since verbal and physical violence is commonplace in many families. Rather, the conflict always stops short of getting the parent so angry that the child or adolescent is expelled from the family. Once again Fairbairn understood this reality, noting that if the rejected child dared to attack the parent directly for being a bad parent, the child would be faced with an *even worse parent* who, in retaliation, might reject the child completely.

The most interesting examples of indirect hostility toward a rejecting parent were reported to me by a former patient. He was the son of a successful attorney who was well respected in the community but emotionally sadistic toward his family. My patient was singled out for physical punishment and humiliation, and forced to do demeaning tasks while his two siblings were indulged. The rage in this young boy was enormous, but it could never be expressed directly toward his father, for to do so would risk annihilation or banishment. Instead, his hostility was directed toward his father's possessions, which he masked with his apparent carelessness. His first successful revenge-based accident occurred when he was finally allowed to use his father's treasured rowing scull. He repeatedly begged his father to let him try out the scull, which was a family heirloom that had belonged to his grandfather. After a time his father reluctantly agreed to allow him to use it. At the critical moment when the father carefully pointed to the spot where the son should step in order to enter fragile boat, the young man suddenly slipped, and his errant foot broke through the thin planking. At the time he was consciously contrite and apologetic. He could not admit, either to his angry father or to himself, how much rage he had inside, and he covered it with his guilt and profuse apologies.

Several years later, after another period of pleading with his father, he was allowed to take his father's sailboat out into the lake with his friends. He and his youthful companions had a wonderful time, and he had returned home and was about to sit down to dinner when the marina called to report that only the tip of the mast of his father's boat was visible at the mooring. My patient had "forgotten" to tighten a bailing plug in the hull of the boat, which promptly filled with water and sank. Once again, he covered his legitimate, but unconscious, hostility toward his father with apologies. Not surprisingly, when he began to drive he was only allowed to use the old family station wagon, while his sister was permitted to drive his father's pride and joy, a Jaguar convertible. Once again my patient (at this time he was eighteen years old) had another mishap, a "two-for-one special." He managed to lose control of the station wagon while backing up and rammed it into the parked Jaguar, damaging both cars. A year or two later he was grudgingly allowed to drive the Jaguar, since he appeared to be less accident-prone and the novelty of the car had worn off. His now aging father made him promise that he would adhere to the speed limit, and he readily agreed. The moment he was out of sight he would race the car at top speed. He had taken it to a neighboring city, perhaps fifty miles away, and somehow forgot to release the emergency brake when he started for home. As he raced home at top speed the rear brakes became red hot, but the tremendous wind speed prevented a fire. Walking up the front steps, he was nearly run over by his ashen-faced father, who ran out toward the car with a fire extinguisher. The enormous heat build-up in the brakes caused them to erupt into flames, igniting the axle grease and damaging the whole back end of the car. Once again my patient's "carelessness" had severely damaged another of his father's prized possessions.

My patient was never conscious of his hostility and gladly tolerated the family label of being careless, yet his carelessness had a pinpoint accuracy about it that was uncanny. Not surprisingly, he also suffered enormously from feelings of inferiority, timidity, and hypersensitivity to criticism from his teachers. Although this example is humorous, there is nothing enjoyable about the combination of dependency and hate toward a parent who is abusive. The child's hate has to be disguised, or displaced onto authority figures or those weaker than himself. In most cases the parent is spared knowledge of the extent of the dependent child's rage. Many acts of "senseless" cruelty are done to either younger children or to animals by adolescents and young adults who are filled with unrecognized rage toward their parents.

Once again, this combination of dependency and suppressed rage, either masked or displaced toward others, can be seen in the battering relationship. The abused woman is in the same impossible psychological situation as is the abused child. One of the most interesting aspects of the battering scenario is that many abused women attack the police when they come to her aid during the actual battering incident. Chapter 5 will describe this phenomenon and present two different explanatory models that attempt to explain this unexpected behavior.

Impulsivity and the Search for "Substitute Satisfactions" Impulsivity is another characteristic of both men and women who engage in domestic violence. *Impulsivity* is closely related to acting out in that it is the inability to hold back or to keep one's needs in check. It differs from pure acting out in that it is not motivated by tension stemming from immediate sources of frustration. Rather, it is the result of inner emptiness, and a historical neediness that demands gratification. Impulsivity is often a way of life for both members of the battering partnership, and each excuses the other for this trait because it gives them both permission to engage in future impulsive behaviors. For instance, one of my physically abused female patients described her amusement at her husband's recent impulsive act—he had put a down payment on a car they both knew they could not possibly afford. She knew that it would be repossessed within months. I asked her why she was so calm about his unilateral misuse of their scarce resources. She laughed, and said that if she let him have his car she would be able to go to Atlantic City and gamble. If her husband complained, she could throw the repossessed car back in his face as an example of his wastefulness.

As we have seen, the neglected child has little hope that he will eventually receive gratification if he suppresses his needs. His parents have "proven" to him that they are not to be trusted to come forth with support or gratification, since they have so often failed him. This lack of hope in his parents is often combined with a lack of fear of the parent's rejection of him. The withdrawal of parental affection or goodwill has little deterrent power for the poorly reared child simply because there is not much affection to begin with. The child realizes that he can't be deprived of something he never had. The only source of relief for his inner emptiness are "things" that temporarily make him happy. This is the extreme opposite psychological situation from the well-reared child who was willing to forgo a desired candy bar because a confrontation with his mother would erode the good will *that already existed between them.*

Impulsivity always involves some form of "substitute satisfaction" that temporarily makes the person feel better. Again, it was Fairbairn who recognized this behavior. These other forms of gratification serve as temporary substitutes for the unavailable closeness and love. Typically, these compensatory behaviors include the addictions: excessive exercise, eating disorders, spending and gambling disorders, and alcohol and drug abuse. All these styles of impulsivity involve an attempt to fill the inner void originally created by the failure of the parent to meet her child's developmental needs.

Each category of control problem has developed a self-help group to deal with it (Alcoholics Anonymous, Overeaters Anonymous, Narcotics Anonymous, and Parents Anonymous). The fundamental issue in all these separate groups of individuals is an impoverished sense of self that cannot be controlled in the face of inner emptiness and the normal tensions of life. The rejected child becomes an adult with a voracious appetite for substitute satisfactions that help her blunt the inner pain of her emptiness. Personality disordered adults are "emptier" than normals, and feel more pressure from the leftover needs that are a legacy of their history of deprivation. Because they have no good object, either internally or externally, they have no one to please or disappoint.

The following example of Renee is not one of a battered woman but of a neglected child-adult who could not escape from her rejecting parent. The neglected adult who cannot separate from the parent serves as the closest analogy we have to the actual battering relationship. Neither can get away from the abusive object.

Renee came into therapy because of her obesity. At thirty-five she weighed over two hundred pounds, and her weight gain seemed to be increasing. She was a schoolteacher who still lived with her elderly, demanding, and overbearing mother. Renee would eat dinner with her mother every evening, and would be constantly questioned as to why she wasn't married and rebuked because she could not lose weight. In fact, her mother cooked vegetarian meals for her and measured out her portions very carefully. After dinner Renee would typically retire to her room where she had secreted boxes of cookies, which she devoured until she fell asleep.

Renee's behavior displays many elements that are the result of the structural problems of her ego. She was poorly differentiated from her mother. When they were together Renee could not oppose her and felt like an unwilling appendage. When she was physically away from her mother she often did not know what she felt, as if her identity were missing. She had to remain with her mother because she had been so ignored as a child that she had too few positive memories to sustain her if she left home. She suffered from introjective insufficiency. This is the great paradox of both the neglected child and the abused woman; they return again and again to the very people who damaged them in the past.

A second, learned source of the inability to control needs is the child's imitation of her parents. The child from a dysfunctional family is repeatedly exposed to her parents' strategies for coping with their own stress, parents who, in most cases, demonstrated a lack of control in one or more area of their lives. The child suffers internal pressures from unmet needs, which have turned to pain, emptiness, and disappointment, as well as repeated observation of her parent's solutions to the very same problems.

The Lack of "Deep" Attachments Toward Others

Many character disordered men and women have enormous difficulties in developing deep emotional attachments to others in their lives. This is one topic that makes everyone anxious. No one wants to admit that his or her relationships with others, including spouses and children, are superficial, based on obligation, guilt, or the demands of society. This is, unfortunately, the case, and I have found that the less the person is attached to his children or spouse, the more he will deny or rationalize his behavior when confronted. Lack of emotional attachment to family members is a consequence of the absence of love the individual experienced in his own childhood. His parents did not have a deep emotional investment in him, and now, in adulthood, he cannot invest in the next generation. This lack of deep attachments to others does not mean that the person is not emotionally needy. He will often cling to others in adulthood, but his "attachment" is based on childhood need, not a mature sense of conectedness.

I turn to research on young children reported by Bowlby (1988) and carried out by Zahn-Waxler, Radke-Yarrow, and King (1979). These researchers observed that children as young as two years old would attempt to comfort a similarly aged child who was distressed. The study revealed that those children who had mothers that were most sensitively attuned to their needs were the children who were most active in their attempts to comfort their distressed peers. A second study described by Bowlby, and carried out by Main and George (1979; George and Main 1985) compared a group of ten battered children to a matched group of nonbattered children in the one- to three-year-old range. This study found that there were significant differences between the two groups in terms of hostility toward others:

> Not only did the abused toddlers assault other children twice as often as the controls, but five of them assaulted or threatened to assault an adult, behavior seen in none of the controls. In addition the abused toddlers were notable for a particularly disagreeable type of aggression, termed "harassment." This consists of malicious behavior which appears to have the sole intent of making the victim show distress. (Bowlby 1988:90–91)

The abused toddlers also showed no comfort-giving behavior toward distressed toddlers in the group, though five of the ten controls (nonabused children) did attempt to comfort their distressed peers. Interestingly, an exact analogy to the harassment behavior seen by Bowlby in toddlers exists to behaviors seen in male batterers. The adult abuser may start with harassing behaviors toward his partner-victim just before the physical assault begins. The abuser usually singles out a behavior in his partner that annoys him, though in fact he is looking for any excuse to discharge rage on his wife-victim. To my great surprise a number of women reported that their husbands have chosen to criticize their dishwashing technique. The abuser will corner his wife in the kitchen and "demonstrate" how he wants the job done. He may smash those dishes she has washed improperly for dramatic effect. He will then usually close in on his partner and yell at her while she frantically tries to comply with his violent and incoherent demands. Sometimes her distress is enough to placate him; in other cases it is the prelude to a physical assault. The abuser's relief at his partner's distress stems from a primitive form of projection. He initially begins the interaction because he experiences undifferentiated rage and tension in his inner world that he cannot metabolize. When he begins to harass his wife she shows signs of intense distress, and her agitation relieves his inner chaos; she then "contains" the tension that he formerly experienced in himself. This scenario is only possible when the partners are poorly differentiated from each other, and emotions move freely from one to the other.

Bowlby's studies of children remove the speculation from the often made observation that abusive adults come from families where abuse was shown to them in childhood. The greatest value of these studies is that they are able to demonstrate the effects of lack of parental attachment on children as young as two years of age, and link early childhood patterns of behavior with similar behaviors seen in adulthood.

The following clinical example from my practice illustrates the close connection between lack of caring in the parent's history with lack of concern for her own child:

I was called by a local attorney one afternoon and asked if I would sign a paper for the court stating that I would treat Karen, a former patient of mine who had left therapy several years before. Karen was in court because her six-year-old son had been found wandering miles from home in his nightclothes and had been placed in the temporary custody of the state social service agency. Karen had come to me several years earlier because of severe marital problems, including two incidents of being beaten by her husband, a jealous and poorly controlled man. The moment her marriage to her husband was dissolved, she terminated treatment because she felt that her problems had been solved. Like many personality disorders, she believed that all her problems were outside herself. As we began our work the second time, it became clear that Karen's neglect of her son was a continuation of her own childhood experience, which was one of almost complete chaos. Even though her father was a prominent physician, there was no regular mealtime in her childhood home. Frozen pizza and a soft drink would suffice for breakfast, lunch, or dinner. As a teenager Karen did not have a bedroom of her own because she had angrily refused to keep hers clean. Instead she slept on the living room sofa, an arrangement that she grew to like, because she could slip out of the house easily without being caught. In adulthood she could not remember being upset by this arrangement, and in fact it seemed perfectly fine to her. Her father gambled extensively, and Karen frequently came home and found that furniture had been sold to pay her father's debts. Karen's mother was as chaotic as her husband. During the early years of the women's movement she decided to prove her emancipation from her husband by going on an all-women cross-country bicycle trip, abandoning her three children (Karen was eight years old at the time) to her chronically irresponsible husband. In fact, she told Karen that she was undertaking this adventure for Karen's benefit. Karen was supposed to see how strong her mother could be and use that as an example to emulate in her own life. Rather than strengthening Karen, it eroded her already damaged sense of self and reduced her trust in, and attachment to, others. She experienced her mother's abandonment of her as a statement that she (Karen) wasn't worth nurturing. During her adolescence, Karen's two older siblings lived partially on their own and partially at "home," often arriving at dinnertime in hope that a meal was being served. Like Karen, the two older children felt that this lifestyle was perfectly natural and did not experience overt anger or resentment toward their neglectful parents. As an adult Karen designed restaurant interiors for a living as a consultant; she was unable to tolerate the discipline of working for others for any length of time. She would often begin work late in the afternoon and discover that the sun had come up the next morning. Her house was littered with items she had bought that failed to hold her interest. Some were not even unwrapped. Her chaotic style also involved money. She had no credit, for she would spend her credit cards up to the limit on items that caught her eye for the moment but meant nothing to her later on. When I confronted Karen about her neglect of her son, she justified her lack of care by saying that it was teaching him to be more independent—the same position that her mother took during her childhood.

Karen is typical of many chaotic but not overly hostile character disorders who have experienced neglect rather than abuse. She never internalized rules, self-regulation, or developed emotional attachments to others because her parents were emotionally indifferent to her. As an adult she drifted through life, indifferent to the needs of her child. The lack of attachment in her original family left her unable to develop deep attachments to either her son or to adult partners. Like many interpersonally cold individuals, Karen denied her lack of connection with fervor and insisted that she was "extremely close" to her son. Lack of deep emotional ties to others plays an important role in the battering scenario. Mature adults who had deep emotional attachments to their parents during childhood are simply not capable of physical abuse of a loved partner. Harry Harlow, the preeminent animal researcher of the modern era, did dozens of carefully controlled studies in which he separated infant rhesus monkeys from their mothers at birth. Over the course of his lifetime of experimentation with emotional bonding, the effects of abandonment and the consequent emergence of aggression in his animal subjects he concluded:

> The natural and normal responses to affectionate stimuli are the antithesis of those to aggressive stimuli. The world within us and without guarantee that, given the choice, we will love before we can hate. Anger is often improperly thought to be an emotion pre-potent over love, but this is a result of the fact that psychologists have published many papers on aggression and few on love. If early, antecedent affectional responses occurred, they would establish strong ties which limit and preclude the possibility of incipient, intense aggression. To paraphrase Oscar Wilde:

> > The love or loves that we felt first
> > Will bind our hearts together
> > And afterwards for best or worst
> > These loves will last forever.

> > We cannot kill the ones we love
> > Or those loved by our mother.
> > A hatred cannot come above
> > Our loves for one another.

> Primates either love early or they are apt to hate forever.
> (Harlow 1986:310)

This extraordinary quote summarizes Harlow's life work. He came to exactly the same conclusion that Fairbairn reached after working in the foundling home in Scotland. Both men saw that the early lack of love from the parents (animal or human) was the source of later aggression and rage. When this finding is applied to the battering scenario, it supports the reality that only the individual who was not initially loved is capable later in life of attacking, maiming, or even killing his partner.

Paradoxically, many partners that are involved in domestic abuse seem, at least at times, to be intensely close. However, the apparent closeness is actually a *ferocious dependency*, which is not the same as a mature emotional attachment based on love. It is quite common for these intensely dependent relationships to break up suddenly, because one partner or the other finds a someone who meets his or her dependency needs more fully. Lack of emotional attachment combined with ferocious, infantile dependency accounts for much of the callousness one sees in characterological relationships.

Leonard Shengold, author of the dramatically titled book *Soul Murder*, explores the issue of parents who lack appropriate emotional attachment to their children. His book describes the effects of early neglect on a number of famous writers, including Dickens, Kipling, and Chekhov. Shengold uses the phrase "the undeveloped heart," from the English author E. M. Forster, in his description of adults who, because of their own upbringing, are abusive and violent to the next generation:

> Forster was describing the inability to care enough about another person, a deficiency of the capacity for love, joy and empathy. This impoverishment of the soul is both the result and the cause of soul murder; it can evoke in the deprived and frustrated child a terrible intensity of rage that can burst into actual murder if it is not frozen by isolating defenses. And the parent's undeveloped heart can of course be expressed not only by indifference to the child but also by hatred and cruelty. (Shengold 1989:182)

This quotation links the previously described hate and rage in the abandoned child with parental neglect. It applies directly to the previously mentioned "youthful" offender from chapter 1 who was jailed for molesting and physically abusing his nieces. The deprivation he experienced from his early rejection remained visible in his behavior, evidenced by his thumb sucking, while the rage from his childhood deprivation now poured out on those weaker than himself.

Excessive Dependency on External Objects

I have pointed to the issue of extreme dependency on others as one of the major characteristics of the adult personality disorder. This characteristic is based on the previously mentioned lack of positive introjects. This lack of introjects leads to two separate problems in adulthood: a weak sense of self and an inability to soothe oneself when hurt or frightened.

Weak Identity Before we begin our discussion of the issue of identity, we must first define our terms. The ego has already been defined as a a set of functions, strategies, and plans as well as a storehouse of "views" of the self (and of objects) that the child has picked up from interactions with his parents. The package of views that develops in the child's interior world is a consequence of his parents' reactions to him. Over time this collection of "reflected appraisals" becomes the child's sense of self, or his identity (I will use the terms as synonymous). Thus, the child's developing identity is a small part of his larger ego. One's identity is like a huge card catalog of statements about the self, such as: I am male or female, intelligent or stupid, worthy or worthless, loved or ignored, and trusted or mistrusted. It contains both conscious and unconscious "representations" (memories and opinions) of who the person is in relationship to other members of the family.

But what does a sense of self DO? In effect the individual's sense of self is a yardstick that is used to measure, identify, and relate to the outer world. We know others in relation to ourselves: how similar or different they are in relation to us, how their emotionality functions similarly or differently from our own, what makes them anxious compared to what makes us anxious, what they know compared to what we know, what they think and feel about things compared to ourselves. One can immediately see that an unstable or shifting sense of self will leave the individual in a perpetually confused and frightened state. A simple analogy to a weak sense of self would be a building contractor with a tape measure that varied its measurements from minute to minute, sometimes reading 36 inches, at other times 34 inches and so on. His buildings would be poorly constructed at best. This is an enormous problem for the individual because he cannot measure others in terms of an inner standard, since his sense of self shifts from moment to moment. Unfortunately, Fairbairn used the word *ego* to signify the person's sense of self, and that produces some confusion. I will minimize this problem by calling all groups of self-references *selves*, and reserve the term *ego* to mean the larger set of reality-based strategies and functions.

This issue of a weak sense of self has already appeared in the case histories of Carl, the country singer, and Renee, the depressed schoolteacher. Erik Erickson (1950) coined the term *identity diffusion*, which described his observation that many individuals he saw in therapy did not have a strong sense of self; they did not know who they really "were." This lack of identity is, as I have mentioned, much more obvious in the dependent pattern than in the independent pattern. Independents' often manage to hide from their lack of identity by creating personal myths about themselves, in the tradition of Ernest Hemingway. They identify themselves with their possessions, opinions, or hobbies, and create themselves by filling up their inner void with attachments to their chosen fields of endeavor. It may be an attachment to their particular job or to a cultural myth of the self as described in the following quote by Erickson:

> John Henry thus is one of the occupational models of the stray men on the expanding frontier who faced new geographic and technological worlds as men and without a past. The last remaining model seems to be the cowboy who inherited their boasts, their gripes, their addiction to roaming, their mistrust of personal ties, their libidinal and religious concentration on the limits of endurance and audacity, their dependence on "critters" and climates. . . . They bragged as if they had created themselves tougher than the toughest critters and harder than any forged metal.
> (Erickson 1950:299)

The most remarkable aspect of this quote is Erickson's use of the word *stray* to describe the men who use an identification with their work as the foundation for their sense of self. This overidentification can only happen if the individual does not have a firm sense of self in the first place. This act of self-creation is a sign of underlying emptiness since an individual with a well-integrated sense of self cannot push it out of the way and replace it with a prefabricated self. The strength of the identification used by self-made independent character disorders makes them appear as if they have a well-formed identity and hides their underlying structural weakness.

Both men and women who use the dependent pattern are more aware of their lack of identity than are those individuals that use the independent pattern. Dependent pattern women have a particularly difficult time, since our culture channels most of them into child rearing. This identification as a caregiver is not highly valued, nor does it fit for many women who have been severely mishandled by their own parents. What is more, this role tends to isolate dependent pattern women from the outside world, and it fails to provide them with a stable collective identification such as that described by Erickson. When threatened by outside pressure or the loss of a relationship, the independent pattern character disorder can retreat into his identification and hold his tenuous sense of self together. The dependent pattern disorder cannot rely on any particular identification and is more prone to the collapse of her sense of self because her identification is focused on the person that she depends upon, not on a role or self-made myth.

The Collapse of The Sense of Self One of the major reasons that abused women stay with battering husbands is their fear of the collapse of their identity, a far greater threat than the physical pain that they experience during the episodes of battering. In simplest terms the collapse of one's identity is similar to "going crazy." Eleanor Armstrong-Perlman (1991) described the fear and horror of a total collapse of the sense of self that she saw in both her male and female patients. She observed that the collapse of these patients' identities was provoked by conclusive evidence that they had been abandoned by the object they were pursuing:

> The loss of the relationship, or rather the hope of the relationship, cannot be borne. The frustrating aspects of the relationship are denied as well as the consequent rage, hatred, and humiliation and the shame regarding the humiliation. . . . The need is compulsive and the fantasy of loss is experienced as potentially catastrophic, either leading to the disintegration of the self, or a fear of a reclusive emptiness to which any state of conectedness, no matter how infused with suffering, is preferable . . . They cannot acknowledge the hopelessness of that relationship, or that its satisfactions are partial and illusory, for to give up that hope may lead to a collapse of the self. (Armstrong-Perlman, 1991)

This description is similar to the young child's collapse when she is abandoned by her mother—an event that Fairbairn witnessed many times in his career. The "abandonment depression" that I have described is the result of the complete collapse of the sense of self. Like a child, the adult borderline's sense of self requires an accessible parentlike object in order for the person to remain psychologically intact. Without the object, the underdeveloped adult feels as lost, hopeless, and as terrified as one of Fairbairn's Scottish orphans. Without the object, or the hope of an object, there is no possibility of maintaining an organized and coherent sense of self.

Once the awesome power of the fear of the collapse of the sense of self is appreciated the abuses, rejections, and humiliations that are tolerated by women at the hands of their abusive partners are easily understood. The motivation underlying the battered woman's attachment to her abuser is based on his ability to keep her sense of self intact, and this powers her return to him despite the fact that he is physically abusive. I will reiterate this point in my discussion of the battering scenario.

The two following cases illustrate the collapse of a sense of self due to the loss of the stabilizing object. Both examples illustrate a conflict between the demands of the identity-giving object and the sense of self of the victim. The attachment to the object sustains the individual's sense of psychological stability; however, it is purchased at great cost to the already damaged sense of self. The case of Terry illustrates how an abusive object can actually be a group of people rather than an individual, while the case of Mrs. Jackson illustrates the more common pattern of attachment to a single object:

Terry was brought to my office by her concerned parents. She was a strange looking, somewhat emaciated young woman with a shaved head who had experienced a "nervous breakdown" while living with a fundamentalist religious sect. She had been a successful college student who, for no apparent reason, dropped out of college and secretly joined this group. Her parents described her as a perfect child, although I noticed that during the first session they did all the talking for her. Terry, when she did speak, looked hesitantly toward her parents and seemed to shift from speech laced with obscure biblical references back to the "conventional" speech of a college sophomore. It seemed clear that she was taking her cues as to what to say from her parents' facial responses and other nonverbal information. Later Terry reported that she always looked to others around her for feedback as she had no idea what she stood for in life. The all-encompassing embrace of the religious sect brought her great relief because she no longer had to struggle with "making herself up" differently for different people. She was extremely content with the group for the first month and felt that she had found a permanent place to spend the rest of her life. She felt this way in spite of her having no real interest in the religious teachings of the cult. Her breakdown was the result of punishment for a minor infraction of the fundamentalist teachings. She had her hair shorn, and the humiliation caused by this as well as her loss of faith in the cult as a parent substitute provoked the collapse of her identity. The collapse was also partially due to to the fact that her good looks had been a large part of her sense of self. This, when combined with the fact that the cult (the

object) upon whom she depended rejected her was too much for
her weak identity to bear.

My work with Terry focused on discovering who she really was. Her
family had placed so much pressure on her to behave in prescribed
ways that she lost sight of her inner sense of self. Her family was not
only conventional but also superficial. She and her mother never got
past discussions of clothes or hair styles, and her father was absent
most of the time. She had no parental object to provide a model of a
person with a strong identity.

The object to which the person with identity problems is attracted is almost invariably a partner who is, or appears to be, very sure
of himself in order to compensate for his lack of internal structure.
In general the partner who uses the independent pattern is the leader
and the partner who uses the dependent pattern is the follower.
Sadly, the lead partner often ends up being a dominant, critical fanatic who "takes over" the confused and contradictory identity of the
weaker partner:

Mrs. Jackson called for an emergency consultation. She was suffering what appeared to be a collapse of her identity because of the
clash between her two self-sustaining objects. Her husband had
just insisted that they move to Central America to aid in the struggle for independence of one of the strife-torn countries. He was a
well-known radical who led many left-wing organizations, and
was fifteen years older than she. Exploration revealed that Mrs.
Jackson met her husband-to-be while she was an honors political
science major in college. Despite her academic honors she felt
empty and confused and changed her positions on nearly everything. She compensated for her confusion and weak sense of identity by looking for "strength" in her boyfriends, the first of whom
was an ultraconservative border patrolman. He taught her about
firearms and convinced her to carry a gun to protect herself from
the dangers that he saw everywhere. This relationship failed when
he began insisting that she break off all contact with her parents.
Her father intervened and demanded that she no longer see this
boyfriend, and soon she discovered "strength" (at the other end of
the political spectrum) in her future husband. Her husband
demanded that she become a vegetarian, dress in clothes made by
hand rather than by machinery, and read South American authors.

Mrs. Jackson willingly complied with these demands since she felt it was making her stronger as well. However the demand to move to Central America was too much for her to bear as it would mean the loss of contact with her family, especially her mother, on whom she was dependent.

This example is not specifically about battering; however, many of the components that make up a typical battering dyad were present. Mrs. Jackson used the dependent style and her husband was on the extreme end of the independent style. He wanted total control over her and she was willing to comply with his demands in trade for the security and direction that he gave her. The unspoken agreement between them broke down when his demand to move to Central America conflicted with her attachment to her parents. Despite her extreme dependency on her husband, she was unwilling to give up all of her other sustaining relationships with people (including her parents) in exchange for a cause in which she had little organic investment. Her impaired identity was in sharp contrast to her superior intelligence. This extreme disparity between intelligence and emotional maturity is striking in many borderline personality disorders. Her dependency on others outside herself was based on her history, which had provided her with too few positive introjects. As we will see in the discussion on battering, the weaker the person's sense of identity, the more she needs to cling to the object to keep her sense of self from collapsing.

Extreme Dependency on Others Based on Lack of Self-Soothing Introjects. Those unfortunate children who have abandoning or abusive parents do not have enough memories of being calmed or soothed during their childhoods and so cannot calm themselves when stressed in adulthood. In fact, when they turn "inside" themselves, all they experience is emptiness, which results in even *greater* anxiety. These individuals must therefore rely on others outside themselves to calm them down. This inability to comfort oneself is a greater problem for those character disordered individuals who use the independent pattern than for those who use the dependent pattern. Therefore this is a problem of abusers rather than of victims of abuse and it is one of the reasons that men who batter their partners are so dependent on the very women they abuse. They absolutely depend on their partners to regulate their inner sense of comfort, and without their partners they feel abandoned and at the mercy of their inner chaos.

Many abusive men are exceedingly ineffectual in the real world. They are often intimidated by the normal tasks of life, fearful of others, and have few (if any) close friends. Because of their marginal performance in the workplace they do not receive the normal quantity of praise and the resulting self-esteem that comes to those who perform adequately and have successful interpersonal relationships. Instead they are completely reliant on their partners for their sense of worth and power. Many abusers attempt to take total control of their partners, and this provides them with a compensatory sense of power they are missing in the real world. Some use their female partner as a one-person captive audience from whom they demand total attention while they display their imagined brilliance and trumped up success stories. Without this fragile source of self-esteem their inner world would plunge them into despair.

Sexuality is another behavior that helps regulate the inner turmoil, emptiness, and lack of self-esteem that plague many independent-style character disorders. The physical contact and release of tension is used as substitute for the emotional contact that these adults did not receive in childhood. Intense, need-driven sexuality serves as a substitute for real closeness. It channels tension from other sources into a new form, and offers the release for feelings such as emptiness, lack of purpose, and isolation that have nothing to do with sexuality at all. I have observed over the years of my practice that my character disordered patients were persons of "many honeymoons, but few marriages."

It is not unusual for the character disordered patient to experience sexuality as the only form of closeness available to him. For instance, one of my former patients demanded sexual contact with his wife every night. If she refused he would complain, argue, or go into a hostile tirade until she gave in. If, on rare occasions, she managed to evade his demands he would call her at her job and force her to promise him that they would have sexual contact that night. Without daily sexual contact his abandonment feelings would engulf him and he would experience inner panic. His history was so deprived that physical contact was the only way he felt "close" to his now symbolized wife-mother. His sexuality was driven or motivated by lack of an internalized comforting object, and his dependency on his wife to regulate the tension in his inner world was almost total.

The Personality Disorder's Extreme Sense of Shame

Shame plays a major role in the lives of both the abused victim and the abuser. The independent pattern male hides his shame at being neglected in childhood under a veneer of grandiosity. The dependent pattern partner has the same experience of shame from her history, but no compensatory defense. In adulthood the physical abuse that she receives serves to strengthen and reinforce the shame already present in her. Once again I will turn to an example from childhood to illustrate the development of shame in the neglected child:

James came to therapy with severe marital problems, but our focus soon turned to his childhood. He was raised by a depressed and indifferent mother and a passive alcoholic father who worked on the second shift his entire life. There was no abuse or strife in his childhood, just silence, emptiness, and loneliness. His mother was minimally available to him because she habitually stayed awake until midnight to await her husband's return from his job. Each morning James would find his mother asleep on the sofa, and he became used to making his brother breakfast while his mother slept. She was rarely awake by the time he left with his brother to meet the school bus. He never recalled feeling shame until his fourth-grade teacher came to pick him up for a special school trip. He opened the door for his teacher and then realized that his sleeping mother was in full view. A sickening wave of shame rolled over him and he slammed and locked the door and refused to leave the house.

This is a typical experience of children who are neglected. They are ashamed of themselves for being neglected because the neglect by their treasured parent is a statement to the whole world that they are not worthy of care. The child's self-shame is the result of feeling so worthless that *even his own mother will not take care of him.* It is, after all, one thing to be degraded by a stranger who cares nothing for you and quite another to be degraded by one's own mother. The prior example of James illustrates the fact that the child tries to keep his awareness of feelings of shame repressed. When he viewed, from the perspective of his teacher, the typical morning scene in which his needs were obviously being ignored by his sleeping mother, his shame erupted into his awareness.

The second important source of shame comes from the neglected child's embarrassment and humiliation when she offers her love to her mother and it is ignored or devalued. The best analogy to this form of humiliation is the often dramatized scenario where a young man or young woman prepares for his or her first date. He or she is filled with expectation, pride, and excitement, and spends considerable time preparing for the big event, only to be stood up at the last possible moment. All hope and expectation are openly expressed by the elaborate preparations, and the rejection makes a mockery of the young person's needs. The result is humiliation, embarrassment, rage, and shame. Such is the fate of the young child who offers his pure love to a treasured parent if it is ignored or brushed aside. The sense of self is severely devalued by this repeated humiliation. If this scenario is repeated in childhood, the child will accept devaluation of his love as normal and in adulthood will continue to accept similar devaluations.

The battering relationship reveals an almost exact replication of this childhood scene. The abused woman often makes major sacrifices to please her desperately needed partner. Despite her heartfelt efforts, her partner may reject, demean, and mock them, thus humiliating the abused woman enormously. Even after these repeated humiliations the abused woman does not give up on her partner, but rather redoubles her efforts to please him. The abused woman uses a defense mechanism (which Fairbairn discovered in 1943, calling it the "moral defense against bad objects") to keep from seeing that her partner's devaluation of her efforts is not her fault but rather the consequence of his hostility and limitations. The abused woman assumes that her faulty performance is to blame for these rejections, and this form of self-blaming is a third major source of shame. The moral defense will be discussed in detail in chapter 4.

Defensive Behaviors That Hide the Shameful Self. The extreme sense of shame in their "self" causes character disordered individuals to hide from others. They are so fearful of exposure that they try to accommodate everyone. Rather than admit that they cannot perform a given task they will agree to do it in order to hide the reality that it is beyond their skills. This temporary avoidance of shame has long-term consequences that were not originally considered. For instance, a former patient of mine went for a job interview for a position as an executive secretary. She was turned down for that job but offered a lesser position as a file clerk, which she accepted. Her enormous historical shame made her unable to admit to her husband that she had been offered the lesser job, and she began systematically augmenting her salary from their savings account to continue the charade. Her husband found out, rather dramatically, when their seriously depleted savings account statement came across his desk.

Similarly, the character disordered adult who is asked a question to which he does not know the answer prefers to keep his ignorance (and shameful self) hidden if possible. I once taught briefly at an "alternative" college that had no academic standards or rules of behavior, and offered little if any education to its students. Naturally it attracted hordes of character disorders, both faculty and students. One of the practices of this self-proclaimed college was the students' presentation of their semester projects to their fellow students and the faculty. I was asked to sit in on a presentation by a classic independent pattern character disorder who had completed a semester studying abnormal psychology. It was painfully clear that this apparently confident young man knew nothing about the subject. His presentation was given with the sureness of an authority in the field—as if he were producing definitive new insights into the world of abnormal psychology. I asked him to differentiate the diagnostic categories of multiple personality from catatonic and paranoid schizophrenia. He confused them completely, and instead of acknowledging that he was lost insisted that his confused presentation represented new truths that the field had not yet acknowledged. The audience became embarrassed for him as his discomfort (disguised by grandiosity) became increasingly apparent. Undeterred, I continued my line of questioning, and my persistence enraged him, since his "knowledge" had never been challenged before in his college career. His seeming sureness and grandiosity broke down when he was unable to distinguish neurosis from psychosis, and he left the room shouting that he was no longer going to take academic "harassment." This sort of performance is typical of the severely damaged independent pattern character disorder. This young man could not allow his ignorance to be exposed, for the humiliation would destroy his already damaged sense of self. Instead, he attempted to hide his fear behind a veneer of sureness and superiority. When challenged there was nowhere to hide, and he had to explode into rage and flee the interpersonal field. Had this young man been challenged at home by his girlfriend or partner, a very different, perhaps violent scenario might have ensued.

Another technique used by many character disorders to keep their shameful self at bay is to surround themselves with expensive items. This helps to combat their feeling of envy of others who seem to be fulfilled by the ordinary events and interactions of life. One particular patient relieved her sense of shame by shopping for expensive clothing that *proved* she was significant. She would return home with her new purchases, relieved of anxiety. The temporary gratification provided by the purchases would decrease rapidly over the next few days. Simultaneously the reality of increased debt would intrude into her awareness when she ran across the charge slips. This reality would cause her tension to increase once again, and she would begin planning another shopping trip. The pattern of avoidance, followed by tension build-up, followed by acting out, is commonly seen as the addiction cycle. However *addiction* is not an explanatory concept (even though it has been used as one), but rather a descriptive one. That is, the concept of addiction offers no theory about the internal state or psychological structures of the individual who engages in this style of behavior. These behaviors are a consequence of a poorly formed ego and an impaired sense of self that has to rely on acting out to reduce tension.

Shame and the Avoidance of Responsibility. Another result of the deep shame experienced by personality disordered individuals is their inability to face responsibilities that others take in stride. They do not feel strong, important, or worthwhile, and the normal challenges of life intimidate them. I was surprised to learn that a large number of characterologically impaired individuals do not pay their taxes. This blatant avoidance usually begins innocently enough when the individual becomes excessively frustrated with, and fearful of, the complexity of the tax forms. Instead of facing the inevitable reality of paying taxes, he puts it out of his mind. The next year he faces more difficulties and is doubly avoidant, for not only is he sure that he cannot cope with the tax forms but he also faces the prospect of getting caught for his past transgressions if he does file. This fear motivates him to skip filing the next year. And so it goes, year after year. Similarly, a number of my patients have reported over the years that they would throw away bills that could not be paid in the hope that somehow the debt would just go away.

Avoidance of adult responsibility plays a major role in the relationships of couples who are caught in the battering cycle. As mentioned previously, many abusers are ineffectual in the real world, and compensate for their sense of weakness by controlling their partner. They often demean their partner's attempts to do normal life tasks and take over more and more of the jobs that once brought their partner in contact with the outside world. The more they isolate their partner from outside influences, the more secure they feel, since they have greater leverage to control and abuse their nearly captive partner. For instance, the abusive husband will take over all the banking, food shopping, and even prevent his wife from driving. Over time the abused woman feels more avoidant and less capable of doing the tasks that she once did with relative ease. She gradually loses all her interpersonal contacts, and thus cannot be influenced by their often corrective view of her plight. The abused woman allows this decrease in her functionality to happen because she is motivated by powerful unconscious gratifications that are linked to her passive and dependent role. As her autonomy and compentency decrease she regresses to a position of total dependence on her increasingly parentlike partner. This regressive position appeals to the undernurtured woman's need to be taken care of, and her increased incompetence transforms her into a helpless infant. This is a pathological way of "making up" for the nurturance that she missed during her development. Sadly, it comes at an extremely high cost to her autonomy. The battered woman will resist this interpretation if she is confronted, since it is extremely unflattering. However, if the batterer suddenly leaves she will find that the ordinary tasks of life are now impossible to face.

The reader may wonder why the therapist doesn't insist that the patient "face reality" or put her "nose to the grindstone" and get back into the flow of life. This is a prescription for disaster, because these women feel so empty, fearful, and impoverished that they do not experience themselves as able to face up to any responsibility without collapsing. They have been so demeaned, rejected, punished, and humiliated that there is no "person" within them to face up to anything. Moreover, many battered women do not want to give up the infantile gratifications that they "enjoy" as a consequence of their regressed position. The therapist might as well demand that an eight-year-old child selling lemonade on the street corner go off and run a restaurant. The "person" is simply not developmentally ready to take on the task.

Summary

This chapter has described the overt behaviors that are the consequences of ego immaturity and identity problems. It was designed to give the reader a view of how problems in the ego structure that include lack of differentiation, insufficient positive introjects, and an inability to integrate good and bad objects into a single image translate into observable behavior. The battering scenario occurs in the context of many other problems, all of which stem from the malformed personalities of the participants.

The first topic of the chapter was the independent and dependent patterns that most character disordered individuals adopt, roles that look very different on the outside but that are similar when the inner dynamics are understood. Interestingly, men and women personality disorders can adopt either the independent or the dependent pattern, though most males adopt the independent pattern and most females adopt the dependent pattern. Then four major categories of observable characterological behavior were described, beginning with low tolerance for frustration. This first major category of behavior is based on an inability to metabolize anxiety and chaos in the inner world, and results in the acting out of tension. The lack of positive introjects coupled with a distrust of interpersonal relationships results in the search for substitute satisfactions. The second characteristic of many character disorders is politically delicate, as people are uncomfortable admitting that they are fundamentally unattached emotionally to members of their own family, including their children. This sad admission is the legacy of emotional abandonment during their own childhoods. The third observable characteristic of personality disorders is extreme dependency on others, due either to a lack of a firm identity or to a lack of self-soothing introjects. Generally more individuals who use the dependent pattern suffer from weak identities because our culture helps independent pattern users to identify with their jobs and organizations. Conversely, more independents seem to suffer from an inability to soothe themselves and to replenish their self-esteem. They depend entirely on their partners to perform these tasks, which are necessary for the continued functioning of their inner world. The last group of behaviors described are motivated by shame and include extreme defensiveness and an inability to face up to the normal responsibilities of life.

All of these characteristics are based on ego-self dysfunctions, and are present in the lives of individuals who are involved in the battering scenario. In the next chapter I will describe the two major defenses used by members of the battering dyad.

.

CHAPTER FOUR

The Two Defenses
of the Abused Woman:
The Moral Defense
Against Bad Objects
and the Splitting Defense

This chapter will examine the two major defenses that battered women use to remain attached to their abusive partners. These two defenses are developed in childhood in response to neglect and abuse from the original parents. As we continue the discussion I will present more examples involving battering than have been discussed up to this point. All the characteristics found in personality disordered individuals, described in chapters 2 and 3, can be seen in the background of these more disturbed individuals, and more self-destructive attachments to bad objects will dominate the clinical examples in this chapter.

The Discovery of the Moral Defense Against Bad Objects

As mentioned in chapter 3, shame plays a very large role in the development of character disorders. Two sources of shame have already been discussed: the child's shame that he is not being cared for and the shame and sense of worthlessness from the rejection of his innocently offered love. There is a third source of shame, and it is the result of the child's attempt to "explain" to himself the reason for the abuse or neglect he is receiving. Fairbairn was very interested in the shame he observed in the abused children in his care, and he questioned them about their parents. Keep in mind that these children came from families in which alcoholism, lack of education, and violence were commonplace. He noticed, much to his surprise, that these children could not under any circumstance admit that their parents were brutal, unfair, and bad parents. Conversely, these very children were deeply ashamed of themselves because they (mistakenly) saw themselves as bad children and as the source of all their families' problems. Fairbairn concluded that this source of shame resulted from the children's attempt to deny their parent's badness by taking the badness into themselves, thus keeping the parents good. He called this defensive rationalization (a *rationalization* is defined as a logical but false explanation) the "moral defense against bad objects," and he noted that these children cited "moral" failures of their own (lying, being dirty, not doing well in school) as the reason for their parents' continued abuse of them. Fairbairn understood that without this rationalization these children would experience massive anxiety throughout their development, and this anxiety would interfere with their desperate attachment to their parents. Keep in mind that these abused and neglected children need their parents *more* than well-loved and emotionally supported children. Therefore anything that interferes with the dependency relationship on their parents has to be removed. The child who uses this defense alters reality by psychologically replacing his impulsive and chaotic parents with good parents who only punish him when he deserves to be punished.

Fairbairn realized that neglected and abused children perform this psychological reversal because of their absolute dependency on their parents as well as their need for security in a very insecure world. It is simply intolerable for children to admit to themselves that they have unpredictable and abusive parents, because that admission condemns them to a life of anxiety and a lack of control. A child who is so unfortunate as to have a father who is sadistic, hate-filled, and abusive, and who regularly beats her when he returns from the bar cannot admit to herself that she has a bad father. This admission condemns the child to seeing that her future will consist of an endless series of random abuses from a father upon whom she is totally dependent. This type of future is simply too frightening for any child to contemplate, though it is, in reality, the conditions under which many children live.

The solution to the uncertainty that the abused or neglected child discovers is to assign a plausible reason for the punishment that she is receiving. The reason has to be one that (at least in her mind) is potentially correctible. For instance, she might convince herself that the abuse or neglect is a consequence of her poor performance in school, or because she was slow to get up in the morning, or perhaps because she talked back at dinner. Paradoxically, by blaming herself, the child creates some relief, because it removes her parents from being condemned as bad parents. The moral defense justifies her parent's abuse of her and gives the world that she lives in a sense of order. In addition, it makes the problem of neglect or abuse potentially correctible by the child's own efforts. Once the child relocates the badness from her parents into herself, she can maintain the fantasy that her own efforts might repair the situation. That is, she might resolve that practicing better table manners, washing more thoroughly, or getting better grades will bring her mother/father to love her. On the other hand, if she acknowledges that the badness is inside one or both of her parents, then there is absolutely nothing she can due to change the situation.

This defense gives the child both a sense of control and the comforting fantasy that the world is run by rules. The punishment and neglect that she receives is assumed to be based on her poor performance rather than on the random whims of her marginal, chaotic parents. Once this defense is firmly established in childhood it will be called on by the dependent adult who is faced with rejection from others. Not surprisingly, the moral defense is one of the two major defenses used by abused women to justify their continued attachment to their violent partners.

A Current Example of the Moral Defense

The development of the moral defense in childhood takes a great toll in adulthood, since the developing individual becomes used to blaming the failures of others on himself. This is one of the key reasons that character disorders of all types are willing to tolerate massive rejection from their partners. They simply assume that the rejection that they are experiencing is their fault. Unfortunately, the use of the moral defense adds to the individual's sense of confusion and lack of sureness about her own perceptions. The constant misassignment of blame to herself, along with her defense of others who are taking advantage of her, is a constant source of friction between the individual and her friends. Over time she will completely lose her ability to test reality accurately. The following example demonstrates how the faulty parent reinforces the child's use of the moral defense:

Sarah, a twenty-five-year-old woman, came into her therapy session in tears and described a traumatic and humiliating incident that had occurred during a recent party. Despite her college education and outstanding language skills, Sarah repeatedly found herself with undereducated and underemployed boyfriends who came from a different social class than her own. Her current boyfriend, Keith, had sworn at her and humiliated her in front of their assembled friends for making a party mix that he did not like. On the way home from the party she complained about his treatment of her in front of others. Keith began punching the steering wheel, and demanded that Sarah "shut up" because he was going to really get angry. She continued to argue that her party mix was good, her persistence inflamed him even more, and he struck her a number of times before they arrived home. This type of scenario had occurred before in their relationship. I knew there had been a battering incident when she brought the recipe with her to the session and asked for my opinion of it. This was the third time Sarah had asked my opinion about "reality" issues. Each time the reality in question was that her boyfriend had discovered he could abuse her by pointing to a fabricated deficiency in her. Every time he accused her of a failure she would accept his opinion and search for better ways of pleasing him. She simply could not see that the abuse she was receiving was not her fault. No matter how I tried to reassure her, Sarah would insist that there was something wrong with her cooking, her driving, or her housecleaning. Conversely, she felt that that there was absolutely nothing wrong with her alcohol abusing, surly, and uncooperative boyfriend. Her use of the moral defense in adulthood was a consequence of her history, which was filled with neglect. Her intensely insecure and striving mother had used inherited money and a natural talent as a hostess to impress the world around her with elaborate dinner parties. Before the guests would arrive she would take Sarah aside and tell her that the success of the entire social event depended on her behavior. These "perfect" dinner parties required that Sarah act as the secondary hostess, and she was charged with making drinks for the guests and engaging in social behaviors that were far beyond her chronological development. Often as her mother became increasingly anxious and inebriated during the party she would take Sarah aside and, in a half-whisper/half-hiss, tell her that she was ruining the entire evening because of her failure to make the special martini one guest had asked for at the last party or she had failed to talk to another guest about some trivial matter. In effect her mother was aiding Sarah's use of the moral defense by specifying her failures. Often during the next week Sarah would be ignored by her mother as punishment for her imagined failures and would be forced to eat alone so that she could "focus" on becoming more helpful to her mother.

This example illustrates the operation of the moral defense when it is coupled with introjective insufficiency and shame. These factors worked in harmony in Sarah's inner world, and produced a young adult who was convinced that she was unworthy, and thus easily victimized. There is a very close fit between the moral defense and introjective insufficiency. Sarah was empty because of her mother's chronic inability to love and care for her emotional needs. Her internal emptiness caused her to be increasingly focused on her mother in the hope that sooner or later she would receive the love that she so desperately required. Her acute need for parenting made her an easy target for her mother's unreasonable demands, and she was willing to strive ceaselessly to win her love. Her emptiness demanded that she deny her mother's extensive empathic failures, and Sarah blamed herself for her mothers mistreatment of her in order to preserve the illusion that she had a potentially loving mother. Later in life Sarah's emptiness and fundamental lack of of worth drove her into abusive relationships with independent pattern men who appeared to have the strength that she desperately needed.

Like many introjectively empty adults who use the moral defense, Sarah was never physically punished during her childhood, nor did she come from a financially impoverished family. The moral defense is not unique to the battering relationship. It can be found in a wide variety of relationships where one individual is desperately dependent on another who consistently fails to meet his or her needs. Patients who use this defense today are using the identical defense used by the abused children Fairbairn studied fifty years ago in the slums of Edinburgh. In either case, slum or suburbia, the child or dependent adult has to defend herself from the intolerable reality that she is being neglected or abused for no reason. Once this defense is established in childhood the individual will use it to hide from the reality that her adult partner has no legitimate reason to be abusive.

The Splitting Defense

The moral defense is a cognitive defense that utilizes logic to help the battered woman explain why she is being abused. The second defense that Fairbairn discovered is called the "splitting defense," and it is more profound than the moral defense in that it aids the battered woman's quest to stay attached to her abuser by altering the very structure of her ego. This "structural" defense is used by both men and women, and it was touched on in the example of Sam, the abusive husband who could not integrate the two views of his wife into a single image. When she frustrated him (which was very frequent, given his infantile demands), Sam saw his wife as completely rejecting, and this perception justified (in his mind) the aggression he poured out on her. When Sam became enraged he could neither see nor remember any positive aspects of his partner. The splitting defense is an extreme inability in adult individuals to perceive their partners as containing both rewarding and frustrating potentials. It is the single most important psychological defense contributing to interpersonal violence on the part of the abuser. It also functions to hide the reality of the abuser from the victim of abuse, and therefore plays a key role in the return of the battered woman to her abusing partner.

Fairbairn was the first theorist to describe splitting in the way that we use the concept today. He was initially influenced by Melanie Klein, who viewed herself as a Freudian loyalist and emphasized the child's "instinctual" hate and destructiveness toward the parent. Klein believed that children controlled their biologically based anger by keeping it "split off" from their feelings of love for their parents. Fairbairn had no use for the concept of innate aggression, but he did develop Klein's line of thought about the importance of splitting in the inner world of developing children. He saw extreme examples of the splitting defense in his abused and neglected children, who had been separated from their parents. He noticed that these unfortunate children held two completely separate, and opposite, views of their parents in independent, sealed off ego states that alternatively controlled their consciousness. He recognized that these two separate ego states protected these children from remembering the reality of the neglect and abuse they had suffered at the hands of their parents when they were in the "other" ego state.

An *ego state* is a three-piece unit consisting of: 1. an object, 2. a connecting emotion, and 3. a reciprocal sense of self in the child. Splitting fractures the child's ego into two separate ego states, each of which contains a sense of self and a view of the object. The emotion that connects the self and object in one ego state is the opposite of the feeling in the other ego state. In simplest terms the first ego state is a "good" one in which the parent is appropriately gratifying and experienced as a good object. This good parent is connected by love to the child's good self. The second ego state is a "bad" one in which the parent is experienced as rejecting or frustrating of the child's needs. Under these conditions the child's sense of self is experienced as bad, and is connected to the object with anger or hostility. Only one ego state is dominant at any given time, while the other, opposite ego state is repressed. For example, the child who returns home after school in the second condition will suffer severe anxiety if he enters his house and recognizes that he is "bad" and is attached to a rejecting and hostile mother. He must do everything in his power to repress this view of himself and his mother. In order to preserve this needed attachment to his mother, the splitting defense will automatically limit the child's perceptions to the "all good" view of her and simultaneously repress his "bad self and frustrating object" ego state. The "all bad" ego state is extremely disruptive to the dependency relationship, and the child will (unconsciously) attempt to deflect his anger toward more neutral objects such as teachers. Before we examine the splitting defense in detail, it is necessary to first look at the processes by which the child's sense of self emerges under normal circumstances.

The Emergence of a Normal Sense of Self

In chapter 3 I described the development of the child's identity as the result of the hundreds of reactions that he received, both good and bad, from his parents. I want to add a bit of complexity to that earlier explanation by noting that the infant initially develops many different "small" selves before a larger coherent sense of self emerges. Every interaction with the parent at the outset produces a small sense of self in his interior world. This process may sound strange, however, the very young child simply has not been alive long enough to develop a sense of "me" that remains intact from day to day. Without this foundation every interaction with the parent starts up a new sense of "me." These small separate senses of self develop in response to the separate categories of behavior that the mother (or father) emits. Under favorable developmental conditions the child's needs are met with little frustration. Parental consistency produces many similar small "good selves," which merge easily into a unified sense of self in the child because these separate selves are so similar. The child contains many positive memories that lead to trust, hope, and the desire to control herself in order to please her parent(s).

Conversely, parental inconsistency hampers the development of a single sense of self since the more dissimilar the small fragmented selves are to each other, the more trouble the child will have merging them into a single unified sense of self. Parents who behave in unpredictable and extreme ways leave a variety of small fragmented senses of self in the child that are extremely dissimilar. These selves may be suffused with fear, confusion, or rage—all in response to the same parent. These selves are too disparate and mutually contradictory to merge together into a single sense of self.

Under favorable conditions almost the entire ego of the child is the "good self." The task of integrating the "gratifying part-mother" memories with the "frustrating part-mother" memories occurs easily and smoothly. That is, the early normal separation of the two views of the parent, who was originally seen as either all "good" or all "bad," gives way to an integrated view of the parent. Even under the best of developmental circumstances there are going to be a few memories of frustration and anger at the mother. As I have pointed out, integration of the two separate views of the parent happens very easily when the good memories of the parent far outweigh the few frustrating memories, because the child can tolerate a few negative memories when they are a small fraction of a galaxy of positive memories. When this process is completed the child is capable of *object constancy*, which is defined as the ability to keep the essential view of the mother (or of any other person) in mind even when she is temporarily angry at the child. That is, the child who has achieved object constancy is able to remember that her mother really loves her despite the momentary loss of goodwill between them.

Deprived Development and the Necessity for the Splitting Defense

The deprived child has a very poor ratio of gratifying to frustrating memories when compared to the ratio of positive to negative memories in the emotionally supported child, and so the process of integration becomes very threatening. The threat comes from the fact that integration allows the developing child to see *both the gratifying and rejecting aspects of the parent as parts of the same person after it has taken place.* I will use the prior example of Carl the singer/songwriter to illustrate the problem of integration for the neglected child. Carl remembered his childhood as endlessly frustrating and empty. His mother was often sealed off in another room of the house while Carl was left with his indifferent nanny. He would beg to be let into the room where his mother was working, but was turned away again and again. His only technique for attracting his mother's attention was to be sick, and he managed to produce one ailment after another in a desperate attempt to get her to focus on him. His frustration increased from year to year, and Carl (like thousands of other neglected children) was unable to integrate the two separate views of his mother, since the number of frustrating memories of her far exceeded the few gratifying memories of her.

Carl could not integrate both aspects of his mother into a single view because he could not tolerate the reality that he was completely dependent on a mother who rejected his needs almost all of the time. He had to continue seeing his mother as two separate persons long after he was developmentally old enough to merge the two separate images of her into a single view. The splitting defense allowed him to hide (most of the time) from the crushing reality that his mother rejected him and frustrated his normal developmental needs. If Carl had attempted to integrate the rejecting memories of his mother with the far fewer gratifying memories of her into one perception, he would have discovered it to be like trying to hide an elephant-sized package of rejections behind a mouse-sized package of love. Carl did not have to keep his father split into a "good father" and a "bad father" because the intensity of his early needs was directed toward his mother. As mentioned, his father disappointed him because of his lack of genuineness and emotional coldness. Carl used the moral defense to rationalize this style of treatment by seeing it as his father's way of teaching him to be a man. Each parent inadvertently damaged him in the same way that they themselves were damaged in their own childhoods.

Splitting is a continuation of the infantile process of seeing the mother as two different people, and, in one sense, it can be conceptualized as a lack of maturity. However, the splitting defense is much more than a simple lack of maturity, for it is an *active* process requiring energy, vigilance, and alertness. In effect, defensive splitting acts like a complex psychological computer program that works continuously to keep the child from remembering the full extent of the abuse that he has experienced.

The splitting defense not only keeps the two groups of perceptions of the mother completely separate in the child's interior world but it also keeps the two associated senses of self (good self, bad self) separate. Thus when the mother is gratifying, the child's sense of self is experienced as good, and all memories of the bad self are banished into the unconscious. Conversely, when the mother is rejecting, or unavailable, the child's sense of self is experienced as being worthless, angry, and bad, and all prior memories of the good self are similarly held in the unconscious. The most interesting aspect of the splitting defense is that the memories of love and support in the "good" part-self do not influence, reduce, or in any way impact upon the self-hate in the "bad" part-self. The split between the two part-selves accounts for the fact that adults who use this defense behave erratically both in regard to themselves and others.

These two part-selves act like two different conductors attempting to conduct the same orchestra. When conductor A is dominant, the orchestra plays Gershwin. Suddenly conductor B jumps on to the podium, pushes A aside, and begins to conduct Bach. When one part-self is dominant, the other is completely absent from the individual's consciousness. Carl's behavior in the consulting room illustrated the chasm between his two part-selves. Carl experienced himself as worthless in most of our sessions. However, at other times when his fragile "good" sense of self was dominant, he would feel confident and optimistic, and could not relate to his now repressed "bad" self. Carl, like many others who use the splitting defense, was prone to extreme shifts in his mood because he was unable to "remember" his hurt sense of self when feeling optimistic, or conversely remember his optimistic sense of self when feeling deprived and empty.

The Development of the Abused Self

The neglected or abused child develops a very small good-self ego state since there are relatively few moments of appropriate gratification and support from a "good" parent during her emotional development. These few memories do not produce a strong sense of being "good." When the parent is excessively frustrating, negative, or simply absent, a very large "bad" sense of self develops. This sense of self is comprised of the child's emotional experience of herself as she relates to the mother when she frustrates the child's legitimate needs, either through neglect or abuse. This damaged sense of self (which I have referred to up to now as the "bad self") is dominant in children who have been severely abused, and it was originally called the "antilibidinal ego" by Fairbairn. I will call it the *abused self* so as not to confuse the concept of ego with the concept of self.

The abused self is filled with bitterness, cynicism, self-destructive hate, and, paradoxically, respect for the rejecting aspects of the mother or father. The abused self is the sense of self that is alert and functional during the attacks, abandonments, and criticisms by the parent. The abused sense of self takes these attacks very seriously, and the child develops a deep fear of, and respect for, the rejecting/hateful part of his mother or father. I will use the following case of Jennifer to illustrate both the abused self as well as the suddenness of the splitting defense. As the reader will see, throughout this discussion, it is impossible to describe either of the two part-selves (the abused self or the yet-to-be-discussed hopeful self) without simultaneously describing the splitting defense.

Twenty years ago I began working with one of my first patients, a young woman named Jennifer who had been thrown out of her house by her mother for drug use. She was living with three other adolescents, all of whom came from abusive and dysfunctional

families. They joined together in a pseudo family and all four were
attempting to finish high school. They had similar histories, and
all of them experienced difficulties with controls, which resulted
in acting out of all types, including promiscuity, alcohol abuse,
and shoplifting. In our therapy sessions Jennifer described her
mother as a vicious, hateful, and paranoid woman who had fantasies that she was working with the state police as an undercov-
er informant. Despite the fact that Jennifer had been forced to
leave her home, her mother demanded that she return for family
gatherings, as the relatives had not been apprised of the fact that
Jennifer had been expelled from the family. She was naturally
reluctant to return, and her mother devised a scheme that insured
her daughter's appearance. She would choose one of Jennifer's possessions that had been left behind and would threaten to destroy it
if Jennifer did not return for the family gathering. On one occasion
when Jennifer was late, she found, much to her horror, that her
favorite jacket had been cut into strips and hung on the shrubbery
outside the house. During our first five sessions Jennifer and I
established the "reality" that her mother was a truly horrendous
human being. At the outset of the sixth session Jennifer arrived in
a conservative dress, very unlike her prior appearance, and
announced that she was returning home to her "loving" mother. I
thought she was joking, and made a negative and cynical remark
about her mother's love for her. She contorted her face in rage, verbally berated me for saying such an awful thing, and stated, in the
loudest and most positive terms, "Blood is thicker than water." I
was astonished, and questioned her regarding our "prior understandings" about her relationship to her mother. She dismissed
them with a wave of her hand, saying that she had been angry at
her mother in the past, but now they had made up and she was
going back home. The more I explored this almost unbelievable
shift in attitude, the angrier Jennifer became, claiming that she
hardly remembered anything that we talked about in past sessions.
It appeared to me that I was faced with an entirely different person
than the one I had known previously—a fact that causes many
unseasoned psychologists to mistake the splitting defense for a
multiple personality. Finally Jennifer tired of my lack of acceptance of her new position, and my negativism toward her mother,
and she left the office in a huff.

Jennifer's behavior illustrates a classical example of splitting; she
contained two completely different views of her parent (although

there can be two views of any person) that were nearly opposite in content, and that shifted suddenly. Splitting allowed Jennifer to stay attached to her mother by fracturing the wholeness of her ego. One part-ego (her abused self) was aware of her mother's hostility and hate, while another completely separate part-ego (the hopeful self) was oblivious to this reality. This second, unrealistic part of her ego held an opposite point of view as compared to the first ego. The second part-ego believed that she had a loving mother. The sudden dominance of the second part-ego (along with the simultaneous repression of the first part-ego) allowed her to return to her desperately needed mother without fear.

The splitting defense is extremely powerful because it regresses the adult back to a style of emotionality typical of childhood. It also reverses the individual's view of reality and violates prior understandings and meanings that have been built up between people. That is, prior to her sudden split Jennifer and I had developed a series of opinions about herself in relationship to her mother. We had agreed that her mother had abused her terribly, and that she (Jennifer) was a fundamentally good human being who had been horribly mismanaged during her development. After she used the splitting defense, her abused self was repressed, and this eliminated her accurate, reality-based assessment of her mother. All our previously agreed upon understandings about the relationship between her mother and herself were suddenly lost. The individual who splits off one ego state and replaces it with another is suddenly "blind" to the reality that she saw just minutes or hours ago. This makes relating to a person who uses the splitting defense a very difficult and unpredictable proposition. When I mentioned to Jennifer the aspects of her mother we had previously "agreed" upon, she became angry at me because she no longer felt that those negative incidents were significant.

The Battered Woman's Use of the Splitting Defense

The splitting defense is the single most important defense used by the battered woman. This defense is essential for the battered woman because she has to live with a partner who is potentially life threatening. She must split off all the memories of past abuse to remain in the relationship with him.

Janet came for therapy because her divorce from her first husband was overwhelming her ability to cope. She was a timid and meek woman who seemed to be sleepwalking through her life. During her college years she had been an excellent athlete, and she married a man who appeared to be similar to herself. After marriage she learned that he bathed infrequently, was content to hold marginal jobs while she worked as a professional, and enjoyed living in a primitive, unfinished cabin that had few amenities. Despite her timidity, she complained to her husband about their living conditions. On a number of occasions her complaints would annoy him to the point that he would explode into a rage and slap her until she apologized for upsetting him. Janet finally moved out, after three years of frustration and several dozen incidents of physical abuse. She seemed completely lost when living on her own and continued to live in the same isolated town near her ex-husband despite the long commute to her urban job. She obtained a small sense of security from living in the same town despite the fact that she was extremely lonely and had few friends. A number of months later Janet met the "man of her dreams," a handsome, single attorney who worked at the same company where she worked. Janet did remark that she couldn't understand why so nice and accomplished a man had not been able to find a wife. During their courtship she was greeted by cards, notes, and flowers left on her desk nearly every day. He seemed to be sensitive to her every emotion, and Janet was dazed by her good fortune. As the relationship progressed Steve, her boyfriend, turned out to be an eager, and nearly insatiable, lover, who would show up at her house before work for brief sexual encounters. Without warning Steve was fired, but he found a new job within weeks. He was not clear about the reasons that he was fired, but he was bitter and vindictive toward his ex-colleagues. Janet had just moved in with Steve when he began insisting on tying her up as a prelude to sexuality. She tried to resist him but he argued persuasively that her compliance with his demands would prove her love for him. All of Steve's arguments seemed logical, and she gave in to nearly all of them. Steve then insisted that she have lunch with him because he suspected that his old colleagues were interested in Janet. This was extremely inconvenient, since they now worked several miles apart. During lunch Janet began to feel that Steve was cornering her and keeping her all for himself. He began insisting that Janet agree to sexual contact every night, and he would make a scene if she did not agree to meet his needs. After several years Janet began to sense that Steve had no concept of words that denoted emotions. For instance, he felt that *love* was defined by a greeting card and sexual contact. Janet also realized that Steve had no concept of needs in others, though he was hypersensitive to his own nearly insatiable needs for attention, dominance, and sex. Finally, Janet tired of Steve's incessant sexual demands and began to refuse his advances. These rejections incensed him, and he would become so enraged that he would beat her. Janet actually came for a session just after one of these incidents, and bruises were developing on her legs where he had just kicked her. Seeing my patient just after an assault provoked me to strongly suggest that she leave her partner. She burst out into tears, saying that she might be all wrong about him, that he was a brilliant man who had no faults. I was familiar with the splitting defense and used a series of extremely forceful confrontations based on our four-year therapeutic relationship and my sure knowledge of the character of the man with whom she was living, yet her splitting defense remained intact.

The splitting defense can be absolutely impenetrable. This patient's enormous reservoir of infantile needs required that she use the splitting defense to avoid an abandonment panic. This powerful defense repressed all of her negative perceptions of her boyfriend the moment I insisted that she leave him. Her memory of the hundreds of sessions during which she complained about his selfishness, cruelty, greed, and lack of human feeling evaporated.

The Abused Self and the Battered Woman

I would like to expand on the concept of the abused self using both Jennifer and Janet. Both patients spent the majority of our sessions dominated by their abused selves. They could remember the pain from all of the rejections that they experienced at the hands of their sadistic objects. Jennifer, in particular, had taken the years and years of her mother's attacks on her "to heart," and, as a consequence, was extremely self-critical. This was another of Fairbairn's points—that the child had no option or ability to reject the parents' negative opinions, *no matter how badly they treated the child.*

Jennifer differed from Janet in that she had been actively abused in childhood while Janet had been emotionally abandoned. Jennifer's abused self was filled with self-hate and anger, while Janet's was a void, hungry and desperate. These differences could be seen behaviorally in that Janet was passive while Jennifer was aggressive, caustic, and quick to argue. In cases of emotional or physical abuse during childhood the remembered opinions of the rejecting parent combine together and form an inner object in the child's memory called the "internalized rejecting object." When the individual "hears" the remembered voice of the rejecting parent the abused self emerges to combat the (now internal) attacks. The abused self can emerge either in reaction to memories of the internalized rejecting parent or when "new" people behave in similar critical ways. When Jennifer's interior world was dominated by memories of abuse from her mother, she would call herself a "lying bitch" and feel waves of self-hatred overcome her. These were the remembered words of her mother that greeted her on a daily basis. Jennifer's abused self had a repertoire of defensive maneuvers to combat the accusations of her mother, including argumentation, denial, lying, and counterattacks. The outpouring from Jennifer's toxic internal mother also caused her to drink heavily when she was dominated by her abused self. Intoxication acted as an antidote to the pain of seeing herself in such a negative light.

Surprisingly, there is a positive aspect to the abused self which is this part-self's ability to clearly remember the abuses from childhood. The memories stored in the abused self are necessary for the therapeutic process because it contains the record of the historical abuse that influenced the development of the patient's personality. As long as Jennifer remained in her abused self she was able to describe the primitive shame and worthlessness she experienced when recounting how her mother had pulled her hair, left her locked at home as a little girl, and called her every name in a sailor's vocabulary. Sadly, no patient wants to remain in her abused self because it is a very painful emotional place from which to live. When the abused self is dominant, the individual is plagued by a sense of hopelessness and self-hatred that stifles every move she makes.

Jennifer also used the moral defense, which almost always accompanies the splitting defense. Her mother had no trouble convincing her of her badness, because early in life Jennifer had to protect her mother's goodness and her dependent attachment to her by assuming that her mother was justified in her criticisms. Jennifer's use of the moral defense paved the way to accepting and internalizing the criticisms that her mother poured out on her. The formal diagnosis for individuals like Jennifer and Janet who use the splitting defense as their major defense is borderline personality disorder, many of whom are also the victims of abuse. More women are diagnosed as having borderline disorders than men because of their extreme dependency, while men often use the previously described independent pattern and are diagnosed as narcissistic personality disorders.

The Role of Extreme Parental Behavior and the Development of the Abused Self and the Splitting Defense

Extreme negative behavior on the part of the parent(s) toward the child is one of the two major causes of the splitting defense. Excessive absence, neglect, or abandonment of the child by the parent is enough to frustrate the child so severely that she has to use the splitting defense to continue her attachment to the rejecting object. This was essentially Janet's history. On the other hand, extreme hostility on the part of a parent also guarantees the development of this defense in the child. The parent's hostility toward the child forces that child to split the memory of the enraged mother and the gratifying mother into two separate perceptions. I emphasize the role of the mother, however, the splitting defense can develop in relation to the father as well. Extreme parental hostility produces the splitting defense because it is impossible for the child to see any of the "goodness" in her parent when the parent is in a rage. The intensity of the parent's aggression makes him or her look like an entirely different person to the child. In this sense the splitting defense is based on a reasonable perception of the child's that her parent(s) behave like completely different people at different times. A major difference between healthy and dysfunctional parents is the "extremeness" of their behavior. Healthy parents have their rage under control, and, therefore, always act like "themselves." The child of healthy parents can almost always "see" the love behind the anger. Primitive parents, on the other hand, can become so consumed by rage that they appear to be completely different people—thus encouraging and reinforcing the splitting process.

An example of extreme parental hostility that caused splitting was displayed by a former patient who had a father that lost control of his rage numerous times during the patient's childhood. This young man recalled that at age twelve or so he jokingly called his father a "jerk" just as his father was turning into the driveway. His father, who was still in the car, ran the car up on the grass and around the house trying to run down his now terror-filled son. Under most conditions this man was an acceptable father, however the extremeness of his behavior created a split off abused self in his son that was filled with terror. This patient's abused self was deeply connected to, and fearful of, the internalized memory of his unpredictable and explosive father. When my now adult patient "remembered" the rages of his now deceased father, he often felt suicidal. In effect, his internalized father was trying to kill him once again. Now, twenty years later, my patient found himself behaving in violent ways toward his own son; he was playing the role of his deceased father, and his son was, in turn, developing a very large abused self in reaction to my patient's anger. The emergence of these behaviors in himself, behaviors that he despised in his father, brought him to my office. This is an important point that applies to victims of battering as well. The violence and abuse that is experienced by victims of battering becomes part of their inner structure and fills them with intense fear and rage.

The Action and Expressions of the Abused Self

The child (and later the adult) who splits off large numbers of memories of parental rejection into her abused self is resting on the edge of a very sharp blade. Any little disappointment in her current life can provoke the sudden emergence of her abused self. The sudden dominance of this part-self will cause a rapid mood change. The abused self is not always characterized by self-destructive hate or defensive hostility toward others. It can simply appear as a sudden shift into deep disappointment and resentment. The uninformed observer, who has no idea of the inner world of the borderline individual, may be startled to see another person (or personality) suddenly jump out of the same body:

Sandy came to therapy with her boyfriend, Jack, with the goal of making Jack more sensitive to her needs. Sandy had competed in the Miss America contest and had been a finalist. At thirty-five she was still strikingly beautiful. Despite her beauty Sandy had not been able to maintain a relationship with a man for more than a few months because her boyfriends would inevitably disappoint her. She estimated that since the age of twenty she had been involved in three to four relationships per year. She brought Jack, her current boyfriend, to therapy with her because of her increasing reluctance to venture back into the "meat market," as she put it. She felt that Jack was the most aware of her boyfriends and therefore the relationship held some promise. Sandy perceived herself as being perfectly normal and was not bothered by the fact that nearly sixty men over a period of fifteen years had failed to meet her expectations. Jack was an affable and handsome fellow who was obviously pained by Sandy's harsh accusations of him. For example, he described his problems with her by reviewing his preparations for her last birthday. He knew how upset she became if everything was not perfect. He had arranged for a limousine and driver to take them to dinner at a posh restaurant and ordered a dozen yellow roses. Upon seeing the yellow roses Sandy immediately became angry at Jack, because they reminded her of the roses she held when she lost the Miss America contest. She then took issue with his choice of a restaurant, saying that the service there was too impersonal. By the end of the evening Jack was bitterly reminding himself never to take her out again, and Sandy was silent and convinced of Jack's total insensitivity toward her. Exploration of her history revealed that Sandy had been upstaged at fifteen months by the birth of a mildly retarded brother, upon whom both of her parents focused all their attention. Sandy had been emotionally, if not physically, abandoned from that point onward. As a child Sandy became very fussy, as if nothing anyone did for her could satisfy her needs. This fussiness is characteristic of many personality disorders and is a result of their deep disappointment in their parent's inability to comfort them, as well as the resulting inner rage and emptiness that follows them everywhere. An event, a gift, or a bit of behavior that even hinted of a lack of "absolute" sensitivity to her needs reminded Sandy of her almost totally insensitive treatment as an infant. This would activate her abused self, and her whole history of frustration would then come pouring into her awareness. Her physical beauty attracted an unending string of men to her—men who tried everything in their power to win her favor. Sandy's unacknowledged (and unconscious) focus on her infantile disappointments doomed all her relationships to failure. Any little imperfection in the attention that she received from these men brought back her split off abused self.

The emergence of the split off abused self acts as a formidable obstacle to the development of lasting relationships, because each new person is unconsciously held responsible for all the unrecognized hurts of the past. Sandy was typical of my severely deprived patients in that she denied that she had been abandoned by her parents and defended their "goodness" vigorously. She had absolutely no insight that her reservoir of unmet needs came from her early history of disappointment.

Sandy's extreme defensiveness about her family of origin is mirrored by the battered woman's defensiveness about her partner. It is a very poor prognostic sign, as it indicates that the patient needs to keep her abusive partner "all good." This extreme defensiveness often characterizes the initial contact between the battered woman and her therapist because all that she can imagine is the loss of her desperately needed partner. If the therapist implies that the abused woman's partner is a hopeless choice, the patient will feel extremely threatened. The therapist's opinion may trigger a split in the patient based on her fear of abandonment. She will redouble her efforts to repress all the negative memories in her abused self, thus making the therapist's job more difficult, if not impossible.

Another aspect of the abused self, which has been described but not adequately explored, is its hypersensitivity to real or imagined criticisms from others. The abused self is suffused with memories of being criticized, demeaned, and humiliated, and it develops an extreme wariness of attacks from others. One strategy that can be seen in both men and women from poor developmental histories is a frenetic attempt to make themselves absolutely perfect, and therefore above reproach. Women may strive endlessly to be the perfect mother, have the perfect house, or, when they attend school, to be the perfect student. The entire independent pattern, favored by men, is a strategy for keeping the abused self at bay. Many men try to hide from their abused self by playing the role of "expert about everything." Some who step beyond the bounds of reality in constructing this defensive facade are labeled *narcissistic personality disorder* because the self that they create is grandiose and unrealistic.

The Battered Woman's Second Part-Self:
The Hopeful Self

Now that the abused self has been discussed it is time to move on to the second part-self, which Fairbairn called the "libidinal ego." Once again I have changed Fairbairn's terminology and called this part-self the *hopeful self* in order to keep the concept *ego* differentiated from the concept *self*. In my view the hopeful self, and its associated "exciting object," are Fairbairn's most important psychological constructs, as they are the internal structures that motivate the individual to return to the rejecting object. More specifically, the abused woman's hopeful self can only see a part-object view of her abuser that is all good. This incomplete vision of her partner convinces the abused woman that he is safe to return to, often just days after she has been abused. Janet's view of her partner as being a brilliant and flawless man even as bruises were developing on her legs is a example of the hopeful self's blindness to the negative aspects of the abusing object.

Fairbairn sensed the deprived child's anticipation and excitement at the prospect of finally having a gratifying parent, and that is why he called the child's perception of the parent, under these conditions, the "exciting object." The exciting aspect of the parent comes from the parent's promises to the child, promises to take care of, to gratify, and to love the child. The parent holds out promise to the child merely by her or his position as the parent. The exciting object is the part of the parent that the hopeful self relates to, just as the abused self relates to rejecting aspects of the parent.

Every child, including those who have been severely neglected, can remember events when her mother was comforting or provided emotional support. The reality that every parent makes a few positive responses toward the child supplies the germ for the development of this second part-self. These few responses meet the child's immediate needs and give her hope that more gratification will be forthcoming in the future. The neglected child also augments the promises of the parent with fantasies and unrealistic hopes. The treasured memories of appropriate gratifications (or indulgences) of the child's needs, plus the hopes and fantasies, become organized into a perception of the parent as an exciting object. When the parent, or new object, is seen as exciting, the hopeful self occupies the dominant position. It is impossible to say which comes first, the perception of the object as exciting or the sense of self as "hopeful." It is clear that they always appear together, that is, when the object is perceived as exciting, the hopeful self is always dominant. When the hopeful self is dominant in women who have been abused, their violent, aggressive, and life-threatening abuser is transformed into an exciting man who is filled with the possibility of love. This part-self sees the abusing object as a man who contains the possibility and hope of complete gratification. The splitting defense keeps these exaggerated fantasies separate from the much larger package of memories of rejection, humiliation, and abuse that are repressed in the abused self.

I will return to the example of Janet to illustrate just how the hopeful self can displace the abused self when a battered woman calls on the splitting defense. My distress at seeing her just after an episode of abuse caused me to demand that she leave her partner, despite the fact that I knew it was a hopeless demand. Janet's abused self was dominant, as she had just been physically assaulted. My demand that she leave her partner validated her strong negative perception of her partner, thus making her abused self extremely potent. This external support increased the reality of her partner's "badness," which, in turn, triggered her feelings of abandonment. This paradoxical dynamic is the key resistance when working with the battered woman. When the battering incident is followed by support from a therapist, the patient's abused self will often gain enough strength for the patient to seriously consider leaving the abuser. However, leaving him is out of the question, and the very thought of separation will provoke a massive abandonment panic. These overwhelming fears of abandonment will reactivate the hopeful self's view of the relationship with her desperately needed partner. This is what happened in Janet's case in that her panic activated her splitting defense, which was already well established in her inner world, and her partner was instantly transformed from a violent abuser into an exciting and faultless object. Splitting also simultaneously banished all her memories of prior physical abuse, which were swiftly repressed in her abused self. Perceptually and emotionally, the splitting defense, specifically the replacement of her abused self with her hopeful self, placed Janet on the other side of the world from her previously held positions.

The return of the hopeful self to the dominant position is a great relief to the individual who has been experiencing herself from the perspective of the abused self. The hopeful self not only sees the object as exciting, but the individual's "self" is experienced as being "good." This is the reason that both children and adults develop techniques to keep the hopeful self in the dominant position. When the individual is operating out of the hopeful self, they are not plagued by the sense of worthlessness that follows them when the abused self is in the dominant position. The hopeful self is the part-self that Carl, Sandy, Janet, and Jennifer tried to keep in the dominant position during most of their waking hours. Without the hopeful self all four would face unending years of depression, self-recrimination, and despair.

Strategies for Strengthening the Hopeful Self

As the reader can well imagine, no child or adult wants their abused self to be the dominant sense of self if he can possibly help it. The hopeful self acts as an antidote to the pain and despair of the abused self, and deprived children and adults learn specific techniques that stimulate and strengthen their hopeful selves. As long as they can keep the hopeful self dominant, the split off abused self will remain in the unconscious.

During development the neglected child builds up an enormous reservoir of unfulfilled needs. In a ten-year-old, not only are the zero-through five-year-old needs unfulfilled but they are joined by the later needs of a five- to ten-year-old. The ever increasing need for a parent pressures the neglected child into keeping the exciting object memories of either their mother or father foremost in her mind at all times. This is essential, as these (unrealistic) hopes and fantasies of the parents reduce her feelings of utter hopelessness. The child must, by necessity, return to her abusive or neglectful home after school, since there is no other home for her. By focusing on the exciting aspects of the parent(s) and by using the splitting defense to keep the frightening/rejecting memories repressed, she can return home each day with a minimum of fear and trepidation. The battered woman is as vulnerable, dependent, and fearful of abandonment as is the neglected child (whom she once was). She is often isolated from friends and other sources of support by her intrusive and jealous partner. Her acute need for her partner forces her to maximize the dominance of her hopeful self to hide from her fear of returning to him, just as the child uses the hopeful self to hide from the reality of her parents.

The battered woman will try to keep the memories of past abuses split off in her abused self because these memories are extremely disruptive to the dependency relationship on her partner. She will actively enhance memories in her hopeful self to counter this possibility. For instance, one patient who was repeatedly beaten by her paranoid and violent husband brought a wedding picture with her to her therapy sessions. She could not allow her abused self to become too potent because the smallest thought of leaving him would trigger an anxiety attack. Whenever the true horror of her current situation overcame her she would change the subject and refer to the ever present picture, noting how happy they were as a young married couple.

This patient's strategy for keeping her hopeful self in the dominant position employed a *transitional object* to support the unrealistic fantasies in her hopeful self. Transitional objects are usually defined in terms of children. They are the things in the world that the child carries with him, such as a "security blanket" or a favorite stuffed animal, to ease the transition from dependent attachment on his parents toward a state of increased independence. The security blanket that the child carries around is suffused with the smells of mother's perfume, soap, spilled food, and other provocative odors. These smells help the child remember positive interactions with his mother, and these comforting memories allow him to continue exploring the world without running back to her for constant reassurance. The neglected child not only must hide from the split off package of negative memories but also keep his weak package of positive memories intact. Transitional objects act as a boost to the weak group of positive memories and allow the hopeful self to retain its dominance over the abused self.

In adulthood the problem remains, since memories of support and love from the parents are needed to keep the individual from falling into despair. Many undernurtured adults surround themselves with memorabilia that help to evoke memories of their parents. It is not unusual to find that a developmentally deprived adult has gone to great pains to acquire clothing or other memory-provoking artifacts that once belonged to his parents, the very parents that failed him during childhood. In particular, mother's wedding dress, father's military uniform, engagement rings, or other symbols of the family become treasured items because they provoke positive memories or fantasies. Clothing is one of the most potent classes of transitional objects since these articles were actually touching the lost parent. One former patient, who had a physically abusive and demeaning father, had all of his father's suits retailored to fit him after his parent died. These suits were powerful transitional objects that helped him remember his desperately needed (but frustrating) father. His father had been so hostile to him that he had trouble feeling any attachment to him unless he was wearing one of the suits. Once again we see the central dilemma of the neglected child: the less parenting he originally received the more he needs parenting, and his need for it increases over time. In terms of the battered woman the need for parent(s) that she never had is displaced and transferred to her partner, who serves as a substitute parent.

The most interesting example of deprived children fighting over transitional objects that I have seen occurred when I was hired to mediate a dispute among three "adult" brothers who were fighting over an automobile:

Three brothers who had recently lost their father agreed to mediation in order to settle a dispute over the father's most symbolically stimulating transitional object, his Buick convertible. This automobile had become his trademark. The oldest brother had secretly taken the car and stored it in an undisclosed location as soon as his father had passed away. This infuriated the second and third brothers, who had each compensated themselves for the loss of this highly valued transitional object by purchasing identical 1955 Buick convertibles of their own through a specialty car dealer. Despite the fact that they all had the "same" cars, the second and third brothers were seeking "shared custody" of the primary car, the one that had been driven by their father. As I explored the family history it became apparent that their father, a Greek immigrant, had been brutal, self-centered, and ungiving in the extreme. He owned and ran a restaurant, and demanded that his three sons work long hours while they were in school. He dominated and controlled everyone in the family, and went into a tirade when his oldest son wanted to go to an out-of-state college. The father won that battle by refusing to pay the tuition. His son backed down, stayed home, and enjoyed the regressive pleasure of having his father pay for his tuition at a local college. None of the considerable accomplishments of the three sons were ever praised, and their desires to take more responsibility at the restaurant were continually thwarted. Their father had been very abusive to their long ago deceased mother, who, given their description, was probably relieved to be out of her husband's reach. Despite all the negative evidence about their father, these three brothers initially idealized him, and rationalized that his harsh treatment of them had been helpful to their "development." In fact, all three sons were emotionally underdeveloped; all were unmarried, fearful, and contemptuous of women, filled with a deep and abiding sense of inadequacy, and unable to begin life as separate individuals. The difficulty in dealing with them, from a technical standpoint, was to shift their focus from their conflict over the last remnant of their desperately needed father to the larger issue of their shared internal emptiness and their compensatory need for transitional objects.

This is only one example of many that I have dealt with over the years. The developmentally deprived adult must cling to transitional objects because they prompt and enhance his introjectively impoverished inner world and keep his hopeful self in the dominant position. Without family artifacts, these patients may plunge back into the grip of their abused selves. Without the physical reminders of transitional objects poorly reared adults may be able to remember only the painful aspects of their childhoods. Transitional objects are always associated with good (and enhanced) memories of childhood. I have yet to see an abused adult seek out, and treasure, the strap that his father used to beat him. In effect, adults who rely on transitional objects are seeking to revive memories of the loving family they never had.

The Hopeful Self and The Distortion of Reality

The hopeful self is not realistic because it does not have access to the repressed memories of neglect and because it enhances and distorts the few good events and interactions that occurred during childhood. One of the greatest distortions of reality by a patient's hopeful self that I have encountered was reported to me by a woman who was severely rejected by her father, now living in Western Canada. My patient would occasionally write or call him, despite the fact that he was full of criticism of her, and full of praise of her brother. All of their interactions were the result of my patient calling him— he never reciprocated by returning her calls or responding to her letters. At one point in our work, my patient began getting harassing phone calls in the middle of the night. The caller would say nothing and simply hang up when my patient asked who was calling. She was not distressed by these calls, and, in fact, welcomed them, as her unrealistic hopeful self concluded that her father was calling to check up on her! There was absolutely no evidence of this, in fact there was ample evidence to the contrary, yet my patient's hopeful self distorted reality and thought that her rejecting father was calling her. We will see this pattern of distortion of reality by the hopeful self again and again in the cases of battered women who, despite being brutally beaten, return to their abusive partners in the grip of the yearnings and fantasies that are active in their hopeful selves.

The hopeful self is the psychological mechanism that allows the abused woman to return to her partner without fear. The reader might argue that no rational person would, or could, return to an abuser without fear. *However the splitting defense is so powerful that it allows apparently normal individuals to engage in extremely self-destructive behaviors without experiencing anxiety.* Friends and family of the abused woman can see and feel the danger, but the individual using this defense cannot. The hopeful self is filled with unrealistic optimism about the future because it is not tempered by memories of failure from the past. When the individual operates from this part-self, all the memories of pain and abuse are split off and repressed and are thus unavailable to consciousness. The hopeful self is unrealistic, because it is filled with exaggerated fantasies that the abuser will provide all the love necessary to fill up the inner void left over from childhood. This ego state leads individuals with borderline personality disorders into endless trouble as they blindly return to hopeless relationships and are then surprised when they fail.

I will return to the example of Jennifer, the high school girl who was expelled by her mother and then returned home in the grip of the hopeful self. This particular example demonstrates the fragility of relationships based on this unrealistic part-self. Jennifer and her mother had a three-day "honeymoon" that came to an abrupt end when Jennifer was overheard by her mother as she was talking on the telephone. She was promising her boyfriend various romantic scenarios for their next date. Jennifer's mother went into a violent rage, and began screaming at her while she was still on the phone. This soon escalated into a mutual screaming match, as Jennifer's hopeful self was once again split off and her abused self returned to battle with her rejecting object mother. Jennifer was once again expelled from the house and told she would never be allowed to return. All of Jennifer's unrealistic hopes and simplistic platitudes, including her statement that "blood is thicker than water," were repressed in her hopeful self. She returned to the prior cynical and bitter attitude characteristic of her abused self.

The unrealistic hopeful self only exists in individuals who have been deeply disappointed by their early object relationships. Normal individuals do not suddenly develop the splitting defense in adulthood to protect themselves from disappointment in their current relationships. Healthy adults leave relationships when primitive behavior or undeserved rejection comes from the object of their desire. Conversely, when an adult with an intact splitting defense is confronted with rejection from a frustrating object he simply turns to this preexisting defense in order to hide from the aspects of the object that threaten the continuation of the relationship.

Futile Attachments: The Collapse of the Hopeful Self

Eleanor Armstrong-Perlman, who was quoted in chapter 3, described her experiences of working in a psychiatric hospital (1991). She noticed that many of the newly admitted patients were suffering psychological collapses because of the loss of a relationship. It was clear to her that the relationships that these patients described were futile. However, the patients seemed unable to see the impossibility of these relationships because their dominant hopeful selves could not see the negative, rejecting qualities of the persons they were pursuing. Armstrong-Perlman used Fairbairn's model to understand these patients, and she recognized that they had superimposed their hopeful-self fantasies over the negative and hostile reality of their longed for objects:

The currently lost, or about to be lost other has been an object of desire. They had felt "real" in the relationship. But when they give a history of the relationship, one wonders at their blindness. Their object choice seems pathological or perverse. There had been indications that the other was incapable of reciprocating, or loving, or accepting them in the way they desire. They had been pursuing an alluring but rejecting object, an exciting yet frustrating object. The object initially may have offered the conditions of hope, but it failed to satisfy. It had awakened an intensity of yearning, but it is essentially the elusive object of desire, seemingly there but just out of reach. (Armstrong-Perlman 1991:345)

Armstrong-Perlman's observations support my clinical experience regarding the power of the hopeful self in the inner world of battered women. The hopeful self can overpower all negative information about the abusive partner and repress it so completely that the patient has no memory of past batterings. Even the confrontations from a therapist coupled with the reality of constant rejection from the abuser are often not enough to convince the needy individual that they are pursuing a person who is not able or willing to gratify their needs. Armstrong-Perlman notes that these patients remain intact, with functioning identities, as long as they *hold on to the hope that love exists in their exciting objects.* These patients live off the "intensity of yearning" that was developed in their childhoods and stored in their hopeful selves. The psychological collapse of the self only occurs in these patients when all of the unrealistic fantasies are dashed, and they are faced with the reality that there is no object to meet their needs.

Summary

This chapter described the two powerful defenses discovered by Fairbairn that combine together and allow the abused woman to remain attached to her partner regardless of the amount of failure or abuse she encounters.

The first defense that was described was called the "moral defense against bad objects" by Fairbairn, and it is an elaborate rationalization made up by the child to explain why she is being neglected or abused. Abused children cannot face the reality that their parent is randomly hateful toward them. In order to feel secure the child reasons that she is being abused for a "moral" failure, such as dirtiness or laziness, which then justifies the parental neglect or abuse. It is intolerable for the needy and dependent child to recognize that she lives in a random universe where she is not loved, and is being abused for no reason other than bad luck. The moral defense is used by battered women to explain and excuse the abuse that they receive from their partner.

The second defense described by Fairbairn is used by the abused child and later by the abused woman and is called the splitting defense. This profound defense fractures the structure of the ego into two separate part-selves: the abused self and the hopeful self. This defense is automatic, and results from the developing child's inability to integrate the two extremely contradictory parts of his parents (the gratifying aspects and frustrating aspects) into one view. This failure of integration is a defense because it hides the needy child from the harsh reality that his parent is more hateful and rejecting than loving. If the child were to integrate the few positive memories of interactions with the parent with the much larger pool of frustrating or neglect-filled memories, then the picture of the parent as more hateful than loving would be too harsh to tolerate. The splitting defense allows the child to continue to see his mother (or father) as two separate people, thus preventing the small moments of past goodness from being washed away by the larger tide of rejection. The splitting defense once established remains intact, and the adult is faced with a weakened ego because he has two separate and unintegrated senses of self which switch back and forth unpredictably.

The first part-self that was described was the abused self, which dominates during most of the child's developmental history, and contains the memories of past abuse and neglect. The abused self is avoided, because the person caught in its grip is plagued by shame, inferiority, and humiliation. Many character disordered individuals develop techniques to keep the abused self repressed and the hopeful self dominant. Most commonly the adult with a poor developmental history will stimulate fantasies in his hopeful self with transitional objects. These are symbolically laden artifacts from the past that remind the adult of those few good times with the family.

The hopeful self is unrealistic and only sees the needed object as filled with hope and promise. Fairbairn called this part-perception of the other person the "exciting object." When the hopeful self is dominant the past rejections from the person whom they seek are repressed in the unconscious. Their view is unrealistic because it ignores negative signals and past abuses that warn normal individuals to avoid dangerous "others." The hopeful self allows the battered woman to return to her abusive partner without fear since all the memories of abuse are split off and repressed in her abused self.

CHAPTER FIVE

The Battering Cycle and the Victim's Return to the Abuser

We have finally reached the long-promised discussion of domestic violence. All the material discussed so far on ego development, identity, and the characteristics of personality disorders will come into play when I look at the battering syndrome. The reader will also see how the extended discussion of the splitting defense and the moral defense is required to fully understand the psychological factors that underlie the battering scenario.

The Bad Object

Before I begin this crucial discussion I must define what Fairbairn meant by *bad object*. A bad object is a person who is able to stimulate the hopeful self in his or her partner while repeatedly frustrating that very same person. A bad object is not a "bad" person, but rather one who holds out the promise of gratification, yet fails time after time to satisfy the needs of the dependent individual. Thus the bad object has two facets, an exciting facet that promises gratification and a larger rejecting facet that frustrates the needs of the dependent other. A parent who is a 100 percent rejecting object is not defined as a bad object, since this type of parent promises nothing to the infant, who soon gives up all efforts to get her needs met. This does in fact happen with extremely deficient mothers, who fail their infants so totally that the child stops eating. This syndrome is called failure to thrive, and is characterized by a loss of weight and a failure to nurse during the first weeks or months of life. The key combination that "hooks" the child into returning again and again to the bad object is an alternation of promising and rejecting behaviors that, over time, produce the two part-selves (hopeful and abused) in the inner world of the child. Once the child becomes imprinted on a parent who is, for instance, 85 percent rejecting and 15 percent gratifying, she stands a good chance of pursuing bad objects in adulthood.

Jeffrey Seinfeld, a current object relations theorist who uses Fairbairn's model, defines the borderline patient as one who rejects good objects and accepts bad ones:

> The child tries to take in or internalize the good object and reject or externalize the bad object. In the model I'm developing of the negative therapeutic reaction, the borderline patient manifests an inversion of the normative developmental process. Instead of taking in the positive object relations unit and rejecting the negative object relations unit, he takes in the negative object relations unit and rejects the positive object relations unit. (Seinfeld 1990:75)

Seinfeld observes that the borderline patient rejects people who offer reliable, normal, and consistent love, and, instead, pursues those who reject, abuse, or neglect her. This is an abnormal process, a reversal of the "normative developmental process" of accepting love and avoiding rejection. As we now know, this behavior is the result of a long history of interactions with a rejecting parent or parents.

There appears to be a very close relationship between women who are the victims of battering and the diagnosis of borderline personality disorder. My experience over the past twenty years strongly suggests that the majority of battered women, defined as women who have been involved in two or more incidents of abuse, are in this diagnostic group. Many of the women I have worked with had secondary diagnoses such as multiple personality disorder, or posttraumatic stress disorder, while a few others were characterologically worse, and were more dyfunctional than the typical borderline personality disorder. In general the diagnosis of borderline personality disorder is appropriate for most of the women who are physically abused.

The Delicate Political Question: Is the Victim of Abuse Unconsciously Attracted to the Abuser?

Up to now the emphasis in the discussion of splitting has been on the lack of availability of certain information that prevents women (and men) from seeing the full negative aspects of both their original parents and their adult partners. However, there is much more to the pursuit of bad objects than simply not seeing the "badness" in the person. Much of the recent literature on battered women attempts to minimize the victim's attraction to abusive men. This is done in the politically based hope that sympathy can be gained for the plight of abused women if they are portrayed as innocent victims who have no role in their victimization. In fact, the victim of abuse *is inno-cent*, but her innocence is based on her psychological immaturity and the malformation of her ego structure, which does not allow her to protect herself from the abuser. There is little question that many, if not most, battered women unconsciously seek out batterers. The fact that they do *does not make them guilty of anything or deserve the abuse they receive.* Their inner structures are so abnormal that the rules of logic and self-preservation are subverted.

Sadly, there is a long history of hostility toward the victims of domestic abuse, which has led up to the current-day politics surrounding this issue. Once again, Freud's theory has played a key role. The current desire to minimize the reality that many abused women find one abusive partner after another comes from a reaction against a widely held historical belief that women were naturally masochistic. This belief was based on Freud's theory holding that masochism was a "normal" aspect of the feminine character. His theory has been used to support the notion that the abused woman was just carrying out a preprogrammed biological inclination. Freud's ideas were accepted because they supported a male-dominated society. The result was a lack of concern about the abuse of women due to a complete misunderstanding of the psychological dynamics that underlie the battering scenario.

Freud claimed that there were three forms of masochism: "Masochism comes under our observation in three forms: as a condition imposed on sexual excitation, as an expression of the feminine nature, and as a norm of behavior" (1924:160). In his discussion of masochism Freud described fantasies (which could be entertained by either men or women) and hypothesized that masochism was a feminine trait:

> But if one has an opportunity of studying cases in which the masochistic fantasies have been especially richly elaborated, one quickly discovers that they place the subject in a characteristically female situation; they signify, that is, being castrated, or copulated with, or giving birth to a baby. . . . This feminine masochism which we have been describing is entirely based on the primary, erotogenic masochism, on pleasure in pain. (Freud 1924:162)

This quote strongly suggests that women are naturally masochistic, and that the pain that they feel when abused is experienced as sexual pleasure—a statement that few would subscribe to today. It was very easy for the male-dominated culture to accept this position and to view domestic violence as an acting out of the "normal" female instinctual role. The subtext beneath society's denial of the brutal reality of domestic abuse was the belief that the battered woman enjoyed physical abuse, because she was able to derive sexual pleasure from physical pain. Freud's model was used to justify abuse as the natural order of the universe. It was taken out of context, and not understood as a small component of a much larger, unproven theory, but it served the purpose of continuing the status quo, to the detriment of all women.

An Object Relations Analysis of the Pursuit of Bad Objects

The key defense allowing the victim of abuse to pursue her batterer, or a new and similar bad object, is the splitting defense. This defense only permits one of the two part-selves to interact with the world at any given moment, and isolates the information stored in the other, repressed part-self. Let us begin with the role of the hopeful self in pursuit of the bad object. The patient who is caught in the grip of the hopeful self will return to the bad object suffused with unrealistic positive fantasies for the relationship. Typically within a short period of time all hope will be dashed by some form of rejecting behavior from the bad object partner or parent. The patient will then return to therapy in a state of absolute surprise and outrage. The individual's unfounded optimism of the prior week is replaced with bitterness and cynicism from his now dominant abused self. The patient will report that he was *completely* surprised by the bad object's rejection of him. The surprise is genuine, because the memories of all the past rejections were completely split off in the patient's abused self, which was repressed in the unconscious. His return to the bad object was guided by the hopeful self, which could only see the exciting, promising, and optimistic aspects of the partner or parent. The splitting defense forces these patients to operate on partial information, and this results in an inability to profit from similar mistakes in the past. This defense is one of the keys to understanding why the battered woman returns, again and again, *without conscious fear* to a partner who has previously abused her. Splitting operates like clockwork in many patients, and it often frustrates and angers friends of the victim, who are able to see how self-destructively she is behaving. Splitting into the hopeful self (and simultaneously repressing the abused self) keeps the memories of past abuse at bay, and thus maintains the relationship with the desperately needed, though abusive, partner.

The borderline woman's hopeful self is not the only part of her inner world that is attracted to aspects of her bad object partner. Her abused self is attracted to the frustrating and rejecting aspects of her partner as well. The rejecting aspects of the bad object give the abused self in the victim an external enemy to fight and a person to reform. I have seen a large number of men and women go into a depression when they lose their bad object because their abused self is left with no enemy to fight. As children these patient's lives were organized around their battles with, and rebellion against, their frustrating parents. As adults these individuals seek out positions as investigative reporters or as enforcers of rules, positions that let them symbolically continue the battle with displaced versions of their insensitive or corrupt parent(s). One patient had a long history of screaming fights with her misogynist father. Not surprisingly, she married a man who turned out to be as self-centered, and as hostile to women, as was her father. They would get into ferocious verbal fights in my office, and on two occasions I found them still arguing in my parking lot an hour after their session was over. The husband was an air force pilot, and he was killed in a training accident during their work with me. My patient was relieved at his death, and report-

ed that the only thing she missed about her husband was their ferocious fighting. Her life seemed dull and meaningless without her displaced (bad object) father. Her abused self had no one to reform, and,
not surprisingly, she began a new career as an alcohol abuse coun-
selor, where she could do battle with an endless supply of men who
gave her life meaning and purpose.

There is one more level of complexity to add regarding the abused
woman's attraction to the bad object, and that is the particular allure
of the *combination of promise followed by frustration* that was characteristic of her parents' behavior toward her during development.
Now that same pattern of hopeful behaviors followed by rejecting
behaviors is directed toward her by her abusing partner. This alternation of behaviors acts as an intoxicant to the abused woman because
it arouses and attracts both of her part-selves (abused and hopeful). As
we have already seen, the promise of gratification is the initial source
of the development of the hopeful self, and the rejection of the child's
needs begins the development of the abused self. These two selves
"resonate" with, and react to, alternations of promising and rejecting
behaviors from adult partners. Male and female character disorders
seek out partners who have similar inner structures, since the intensity level of both these part-selves is far more vivid than the quietude
of a normal ego's inner world. Without a partner who both stimulates
and reacts to these two separate selves, life seems vapid and empty.
When two character disordered individuals find each other, all the
danger of experiencing their inner emptiness is banished by the alternation of *intense hopefulness* and *abject despair*. This is the basis for
so many pathological partnerships. The character disordered individual may not be able to verbalize it, but she senses that her similarly
disordered partner understands her.

On the other hand, when the character disordered individual
becomes involved with a well-differentiated and smoothly integrated "normal," he must either keep his split-off abused self a secret, or
face condemnation from the normal partner when his irrational and
emotionally charged part-self emerges. I have heard many stories
from patients who became temporarily involved with normal "others" and waited in dread for their abused selves to emerge. In one
particular example a beautiful and seductive patient was being "res-
cued" from her physically abusive husband by the attorney who had
handled her divorce. She described him as a straight-laced, serious

fellow who was unmarried and clearly attracted to her. They became friends after her divorce and he invited her to meet his family in Boston. She feared that if she refused his invitation he would lose interest in her, so she agreed to go with great reservations. She was enormously intimidated by his high-functioning family and feared that they would detect her secret. As they drove down, she became more and more agitated, and began to irrationally criticize his family, even though she had never met them. She reported that she survived the introductions, but began to drink wine at the first opportunity to calm her growing inner dread. The dinner proceeded normally, but my patient felt like she was dying inside, since she was sure that his family was scrutinizing her intensely. She could not stand the tension and brought negative attention upon herself by telling a series of exceedingly inappropriate jokes. This act on her part reduced her unbearable tension as she no longer feared exposure. She preferred to expose the worst part of herself rather than live in the dread that her secret would be involuntarily discovered. Naturally, her behavior alienated her hosts, who then became cool to her. She reported that she felt enormously relieved on the way home, and was eager to seek out people who understood her. I have previously mentioned the "strain" on the personality disordered individual when she gets into the company of normals. This example is a good illustration of that strain, which arises from the disordered individual's sure knowledge that her normal partner will not understand, or tolerate, the abused self when it emerges. Therefore, there is a tangible sense of relief when two character disordered individuals pair up. They understand each other completely, and do not have to hide their irrationally aggressive, and sensitive, abused selves from each other.

Repetition Compulsion: Two Views

The classical psychoanalytic concept that explains the human pattern of unconsciously choosing marital partners, friends, or lovers who reject the individual in the very same manner that he was rejected in childhood is called repetition compulsion. It has two explanations, one based on Freud's original theory and the other based on the later work of Fairbairn. Freud noted, in *Beyond the*

Pleasure Principle (1920), that the unconscious seeks to return to the major unresolved traumas of childhood in an attempt to master the conflict. This astute explanation was a small (and the best) part of Freud's discussion of repetition compulsion. Repetition compulsion confronted Freud with a theoretically troubling pattern of human behavior. He observed that his patients persisted in returning to painful situations that contained no possibility of libidinal pleasure. These patients were violating the most basic concept in his model, the pleasure principle. He was greatly impressed by the strength and persistence of the futile repetitions of earlier relationships: "The impression they give is of being pursued by a malignant fate or possessed by some `daemonic' power" (Freud 1920:21). He could not ignore these repetition compulsions, both because of their strength and because they contradicted the central notion of his instinct/drive-based model. Freud realized that libidinal pleasure had nothing to do with the behavior of many of his patients:

> It is clear that the greater part of what is re-experienced under the compulsion to repeat must cause the ego unpleasure, since it brings to light activities of repressed instinctual impulses. . . . But we come now to a new remarkable fact, namely that the compulsion to repeat recalls from past experiences which include no possibility of pleasure, and which can never, even long ago, have brought satisfaction even to instinctual impulses which have since been repressed. (Freud 1920:20)

Freud's sharp clinical observations started him on the right track. He described a number of case histories, which sound absolutely contemporary, of patient after patient who repeatedly became involved with people who betrayed them in precisely the same manner as had their parents. He had to develop a new concept to explain this contradiction of his pleasure principle, and he was constrained by his belief in instincts to invent a new instinct-based drive. He could not step outside his model and postulate that these patients were recreating their earliest relationships, because that would have shifted the emphasis toward a form of attachment theory and away from instinct theory. This new instinct, which he called the "death instinct" had as its (assumed) goal the return of the organism to an earlier state, that is, to a condition prior to life. Sadly, Freud's sharp perceptions of repetition compulsion in his patients, which started with great promise, led to this concept, which is the most pessimistic and unconvincing part of his theory. The death instinct was supposed to guide the organism to death in a prescribed manner. The previously featured libidinal instincts were suddenly reduced in stature by this new concept. Libido was reduced to the secondary role of keeping the organism alive until it could die in the manner programmed by the death instinct. Freud's clinical observations were clear, accurate, enormously insightful, and have withstood the test of time. Conversely, the psychological model that he developed to explain many of his observations was not up to the same high standard.

Fairbairn started with Freud's theory, observed his abandoned and abused children and his adult patients, and produced a very different explanatory model. He saw that the return to the original bad object, or the attraction to a new, symbolically equivalent bad object, was the central aspect of human psychopathology. He recognized that the child's attachment to its first object is the essential formative factor in the development of the personality. Problems within the original parent-child relationship are repeated in adulthood because they recreate the same style of attachment that was originally experienced. He recognized that repetition compulsion was, in actuality, a return to the bad object rather than an attempt to master early trauma. When Fairbairn's patients returned to their abusive parents, or to new individuals who treated them badly, they were recreating the emotional reality of their earliest attachment. He understood that the histories of his abused children *contained a toxic combination of negative, frustrating feelings mixed in with a small amount of love.* Thus, the poorly reared child feels that "love" is defined by a combination of antithetical feelings rather than by the straightforward feeling of being accepted and treasured by a caring person. Conversely, the freely given love from a normal person is not perceived to be love but rather is experienced as something foreign—something that bears no relation to the experience of love at all. An analogy to the character disordered individual's inability to experience love can be made to certain high frequency sounds that exist but that cannot be detected by the human ear. Like high frequency sound genuine adult love enters into the lives of many character disordered individuals, however, they are unable to either recognize or respond to it positively. In effect, the adult who has lost his "bad object" parents remains symbolically and emotionally attached to them by recreating relationships with "new" bad objects. Real love, to the adult who was poorly parented, includes a mix of antithetical feelings: rejection, self-hate, flashes of hope, moments of passion, intense longing, despair, extreme closeness, repeated abandonments, and others that are less identifiable.

I will now examine two cases of repetition compulsion and compare Freud's model to Fairbairn's. Repetition of the childhood relationship often appears to contain some aspects of mastery, as Freud claimed. However, the larger part of repetition is the recreation of the identical emotional experience of childhood. First, let us return to the case of June, the driven television executive who used the independent style. On the surface it appears that June's adult world was an attempt to master her childhood trauma, in which she was put in charge of incompetent parents. There is some merit to this explanation, if one ignores the later part of Freud's theory, which saw repetition compulsion as the work of the death instinct. However, what Freud's model fails to see is the role that June's first attachment played in the suffering that she later experienced. The emotional recreation of the pain *is the unconscious goal* of June's repetition compulsion. Freud's model sees the suffering as a temporary condition that she hoped to surmount. He had no notion that the patient was recreating an attachment to a bad object, because his theory was, simply, a drive theory rather than an attachment theory. Freud believed that attachments to external objects had little if anything to do with the development of the personality structure.

A closer look at June's predicament with Fairbairn's model reveals that her repetition was a recreation of her experience of frustration with her parents, who did not love her, saddled her with constant anxiety, frustrated her legitimate developmental needs, and overwhelmed her with adult tasks. In adulthood June created the exact same set of feelings in relation with her "bad object"—her business and her relationship with her boyfriend. Her business consumed her with frenetic activity, provoked feelings of being alone, misunderstood by everyone, and overwhelmed with responsibility. Her personal life provoked the feeling that she was in charge of a resistant and irresponsible child-man who needed constant correction. June's mastery of her early trauma (if there was any) is secondary to the recreation of her childhood emotional experience for its *nurturing value.* She continued to look for emotional support from a self-created, frustrating bad object (her job, employees, and boyfriend). She was as defeated and and exhausted in adulthood as she had been in childhood.

When we apply our knowledge of the inner structures described by Fairbairn to the example of June, we can hypothesize that she saw her employees and boyfriend as exciting objects when they complied with her demands, and, alternatively, as frustrating objects when they passively resisted her. The alternation of these two perceptions was matched in her interior world by the shift from her hopeful self to her abused self. Her two part-selves had external objects to stimulate them and thus she continued to use the structures that had developed in relationship to her parents' alternating rejecting and promising behaviors. The example of June is a good one as she gives the impression of a person who conforms to Freud's theory of mastery, particularly when compared to women who appear to be helpless victims of battering. Closer examination with Fairbairn's model reveals that, despite her apparent autonomy, June was as strongly attached to a bad object as are women who are victims of physically violence.

Repetition compulsion allows the adult to live in the identical emotional world as the one in which she was raised. The following example demonstrates that repetition compulsions do not have to involve other people. The next patient I will describe recreated the identical, bleak, objectless world of his childhood in his adulthood, and continued to exist on the same substitute satisfactions he subsisted on during his development. Once again we will see both an attempt at mastery and, more important, the recreation of an emotional universe that matches the experience of his childhood:

Ray was raised in Boston where his father was the head purchasing agent for a shoe company. His father was a workaholic and Ray was left largely in the care of his depressed and bitter mother. She had two children, and Ray unfortunately reminded her of her least acceptable (to her) characteristics—he was short and stocky. As a result, Ray received less support than his slightly favored brother. Ray's father paid little attention to either son, but did develop a ritual with Ray, which consisted of giving him all the change in his pocket if Ray was still awake when he returned home from work. This progressed to the point where his father would bring him small gifts that he had received from various salespersons who dealt with him as the chief buyer of materials for his company. Every few days Ray would be given a new pen, transistor radio, or other electronic gadget that his father collected at his job. Ray reported that he would wait up at night excitedly wondering if he would be "loved" that night by his father. Sometimes he would fall asleep before his father returned home, however, at other times his father's gifts would make Ray feel that he was truly important. Not surprisingly, as an adult Ray ran a mail order business shipping expensive watches and jewelry to points throughout the country. He memorized all the mail routes and UPS delivery schedules, which reduced his uncertainty (i.e., it increased his mastery) about the arrival dates of merchandise he had ordered. In effect, he learned to calculate when his displaced "love" would arrive. He was very exact in his calculations, and therefore he freed himself of the daily uncertainty that he lived with in his childhood. The mastery issue was less significant than the recreation of his lonely, isolated childhood. His adult repetition consisted of surviving emotionally on the same substitute satisfactions that had supported him as a child. Genuine love, support, and caring were not available from his parents, but substitute gifts were. Ray's childhood taught him to give up on the hope of human closeness. He continued this isolated avoidant style in adulthood, maintaining himself on the substitute love he felt when he received his packages.

This example is one of the many I have seen in patients who unconsciously construct adult lives that provide them with the exact set of feelings they learned to equate with love during their childhoods. As I mentioned before, real possibilities for adult love come into the lives of persons such as Ray, but these opportunities are ignored or turned down. Real love is foreign, fear producing, and not understood, whereas the loneliness and substitute satisfactions of childhood are accepted and experienced as real.

An Alternative View of the Victim's Character Structure

The position that I have carefully developed, that the developmental history of the victim of abuse is the key to understanding the battering syndrome, is not shared by everyone in the field of domestic abuse. As I have mentioned, politics plays a large role in the positions that are staked out. For instance, Lenore Walker, author of *The Battered Woman*—perhaps the most important recent book on battering—takes the position that the victim of battering is destroyed psychologically by the experience of being battered *in adulthood*. She rejects the general observation, made by many independent observers, that victims of battering have been damaged by their history of neglect in their families of origin. This "failure to escape" model is, in my view, a political rather than a scientific position, as it avoids the previously mentioned stigma of the victim seeking out abuse, and it also attempts to free the mothers (or primary caretakers) of batterers from any censure:

> Many battered women's coping techniques, acquired to protect them from further violence, have been viewed as evidence of severe personality disorders. These women suffer from situationally imposed emotional problems caused by their victimization. They do not choose to be battered because of some personality defect; they develop behavioral disturbances because they live in violence. (Walker 1979:229)

As we shall see, all the evidence lines up against this position, evidence that Walker herself cites to prove her case. Walker, by claiming that the abused women she studied were psychologically healthy before they were abused, attempts to absolve women from a role in their abuse. This in my view is not in the best interest of the shared goal of developing a model that is powerful enough and realistic enough to come to grips with the problem of battering. Walker's attempt to exclude all women from criticism extends to mothers of abusers. She claims that they are also free of any culpability in the production of children who end up as abusers:

> Much more research is needed before we can reach any definite conclusions about the relationship between the batterer and his mother. Psychology has done much damage by casting mothers in a negative light as being responsible for the emotional ills of their children. (Walker 1979:39.)

The reader has to assume from this quote that all batterers were either raised by their fathers, or somehow became violent in adulthood even though they were well cared for by their mothers. Her goal is to absolve women from any negative role in either the development of children who turn out to be batterers or the development of women who are victims of abuse. In the process, she adds to the denial and misinformation that has plagued this topic from its inception. The battering scenario occurs when two extremely damaged individuals with preexisting personality disorders come together and try to reexperience their unmet childhood needs in relationship with each other. Once again, I do not intend to "excuse" male batterers by noting that they are psychologically damaged any more than I want to "condemn" battered women for unconsciously seeking out abuse.

The Six Psychological Factors That Motivate the Victim's Return to the Bad Object

Here I list the factors discussed up to now that contribute to an explanation of the attachment of both the abused child and abused adult to the exciting/frustrating object.

1. The child's absolute biological and psychological dependency on her parents prevent her from rejecting her frustrating parents no matter how badly she is treated. The child cannot protect herself from the damage that is being done to her.

2. The infant (and the infantile adult) assumes that there is one and only one possible parent, and he is intensely focused on that parent. The more he is deprived, the more focused, needy, and dependent he becomes on that single person.

3. The deprivation experienced in childhood does not decrease with chronological age. Paradoxically, deprivation *increases* the child's need for her parents, or, later in life, for replacement parents. The more the child is neglected or abused, the greater her storehouse of unmet needs. As an adult the emptiness and rage from parental failures are painfully lodged in the split-off abused self of the adult.

4. In adulthood the poorly reared individual is extremely dependent on others, either to stabilize his identity or to impart a sense of inner calmness. Those who use the dependent pattern often rely on their partner's pseudo strength to keep their own identity intact. For these individuals the loss of the object (or the loss of hope of a relationship with an object) can lead to a collapse of the sense of self and to the terror of an abandonment depression. Extreme dependency can also be caused by an insufficiency of memories of being comforted during childhood, and, as a result,

these individuals are unable to soothe their inner turmoil. They use their partner to reassure them and calm their inner chaos. Loss of their object can plunge them into the turmoil of their inner world, with no one to calm and reassure them.

5. The abused and neglected child develops two major *reality distorting* defenses: the moral defense against bad objects and the splitting defense. These defenses allow the child to remain attached to the rejecting parent and prevent her from learning from past mistakes.

6. The developmentally deprived adult seeks out, and is attracted to, a high intensity mixture of feelings, specifically the alternation of intense longing from the hopeful self and despair from the abused self. This attraction is based on her experience with her rejecting, occasionally gratifying, parents, who provoked the development of these two separate and mutually exclusive part-selves in her inner world. These part-selves respond to the alternation of rejecting and gratifying behaviors from others. Conversely, normal individuals are feared, since they do not understand and will not tolerate the intensity of hostility in the abused self.

Fairbairn's model, when taken as a whole, offers a convincing explanation of what he called "the obstinate attachment to the bad object." There is no other psychological model that approaches the depth and completeness of his explanation of the bond between the rejected individual and the exciting/rejecting bad object. The adult character disorder manages to find exactly the same form of rejection, turmoil, hate, despair, longing, and anguish, mixed with moments of intense undifferentiated closeness, that they originally experienced.

The "Cycle Theory of Violence"

The ultimate demonstration of the return to the bad object can be seen in women who have been repeatedly battered, yet return to their physically abusive partners nonetheless. The same psychological principles that Fairbairn discovered in his observations of abused children in Scotland sixty years ago apply to battered women of today. This should no longer be a startling concept to the reader, as the return to a batterer by the victim is psychologically identical to Fairbairn's observation that his abandoned children preferred to be beaten in their homes by their parents rather than live safely in a foundling home. The descriptive model of battering that will be examined and compared to Fairbairn's model comes from the previously mentioned text on domestic abuse by Lenore Walker, *The Battered Woman*. Her description and model of the battering cycle, which she termed the "cycle theory of violence" is currently seen as an accurate portrayal of the repeated cycle that occurs in relationships between the battering victim and her abuser. Walker's discussion focuses on the most common scenario—in which all the batterers are men and all the victims are women. Walker uses learning theory principles to explain her observations of the battering cycle, and, as I have demonstrated, that model disallows discussion of psychological constructs that cannot be measured, including the hopeful or abused part-selves as well as the defenses of splitting and the moral defense against bad objects.

Walker's examination of many battered women revealed that the battering had a definite pattern that unfolded in three successive steps: the tension-building phase, the explosion or acute battering incident, and the calm loving respite (Walker 1979:55). I will first review the characteristics of these stages, next apply Fairbairn's theory to each stage, and finally examine Walker's model of the cycle of violence and compare the results.

Phase One—The Tension-Building Stage

The first phase of the battering scenario, which Walker calls the tension-building stage, is characterized by minor battering events that are either denied by the female partner or minimized in the hope that she can contain her partner's rage:

> She may become nurturing, compliant, and may anticipate his every whim; or she may stay out of his way. She lets the batterer know that she accepts his abusiveness as legitimately directed toward her. It is not that she believes she should be abused; rather, she believes that what she does will prevent his anger from escalating. . . . She is not interested in the reality of the situation, because she is desperately attempting to prevent him from hurting her more. In order for her to sustain this role, she must not permit herself to get angry with the batterer. She resorts to a very common psychological defense—called, of course, "denial" by psy-

chologists. She denies to herself that she is angry at being unjust-
ly hurt psychologically or physically. She rationalizes that perhaps
she did deserve the abuse, often identifying with the batterer's
faulty reasoning. (Walker 1976:56)

This description, as well as others throughout Walker's book,
attempts to substitute observation for explanation. That is, the reader is supposed to use common sense to understand these events, as if
they were self-explanatory and needed no interpretation. For example, Walker presents the victim's tolerance for abuse as if it were a
normal event. She minimizes the extreme psychopathology displayed by the victim by noting that denial is a common defense used
by many people. One has to ask, What is the victim's motivation for
the denial? Denial may be common, but why does the abused woman
deny that she is getting pushed around by the man who is supposed
to love her? Indeed, what is the motivation for the "faulty reasoning"
used by the victim when she agrees that her cooking is not up to par?
There are powerful motivations underlying these behaviors that are
not explained. The basic psychological analysis of most of the events
that Walker describes is that the victim is afraid of her abuser. This
simplistic thesis is not powerful enough to explain the behaviors
described in the very first phase of the abuse cycle. If fear is the motivation, why does the victim deny the abuse? Why does the victim
stay with the abuser after the first incident of abuse?

When we look at this stage from Fairbairn's perspective, we have
a more detailed analysis of both the victim's and the abuser's motivations and dynamics. This stage can be characterized as one in
which the female partner uses both the splitting defense and the
moral defense to remain in her hopeful self, despite the fact that her
partner is behaving in an extremely rejecting manner. That is, the
female partner tries to force herself to remain optimistic and view
her partner as an exciting object, even though he is, in reality, physically pushing her around. Her husband or partner, on the other
hand, sees her from the perspective of his abused self, and she therefore appears to him to be a rejecting object. This happens when the
male partner imagines that his infantile, unspoken needs have been
ignored by his female partner. Perhaps the abuser was frustrated at
his job and could not act out hostility toward his superiors. His low
tolerance for frustration demands that he act out his inner turmoil,

and his dependent partner then becomes an easy discharge site for his rage.

The female partner is motivated to accept the abuse, while forcing herself to stay in her hopeful self, not by fear of physical abuse, as Walker claims, but rather by her extreme dependency needs on her partner. If she loses him as a stabilizing object for her underdeveloped ego, she increases the possibility of the collapse of her sense of self. This powerful motivation forces her to inhibit the unleashing of her own building hostility during this stage. Her rage and hostility from the current incident, and from similar past incidents, is split off and held in check in her currently repressed abused self. The splitting defense explains the abused woman's uncanny ability to tolerate abuse from a partner who has injured her time and time again. It must be emphasized that the victim's behavior borders on the unbelievable, despite Walker's matter-of-fact presentation. The victim's ability to remain in her hopeful self despite her history of past abuse is the result of an uncanny and enormously powerful psychological defense mechanism. The victim succeeds in keeping past memories of abuse out of her awareness. She continues to see her abuser as an exciting object and holds on to the hope that with her better behavior the hidden love in her partner will emerge. This effort on the part of the victim to remain in her hopeful self, while her husband abuses her, places an enormous psychological strain on her during this first stage of the battering scenario. The victim's struggle to remain in her hopeful self is reminiscent of the abused child who ran home every afternoon and looked at the birthday card that her mother had given her years before. In both cases, child and adult, the individual tries to force herself to remain in the hopeful self in order to preserve the relationship with the rejecting object.

The abused woman's motivation to remain in her hopeful self is extreme. As Armstrong-Perlman has pointed out, the loss of the object is experienced as a catastrophe that has the potential to collapse the entire sense of self, and, therefore, the abused woman has to use both the splitting defense and the moral defense to remain attached to her partner during this phase of the battering cycle. The moral defense is used to rationalize her dependent attachment to her violent, disturbed, and ungiving partner. It protects her from the reality of her partner's "badness" in the exact manner that it protected Fairbairn's beaten children from the "badness" of their parents. The moral defense also gives both the abused child and the beaten wife the illusion of control. In the case of adults, the battering victim may reason that if she had only cooked a better meal her partner would not have overturned the dining room table in a rage. The moral defense acts to reassure the victim that her partner is behaving relatively normally, because it supports the notion that she is "morally" imperfect and deserving of the abuse. Thus, the abuser's "badness" is accepted by his dependent partner, and he is not perceived to be as "bad" as his behavior indicates.

I have seen an analogy to the first stage in the battering cycle in delinquent young men who also had to inhibit their aggression toward their physically abusive but desperately needed fathers. I was asked to do psychological examinations on a number of teen-age boys who had been arrested for various offenses, including unprovoked attacks on police officers. These young men were later referred to me through probation and parole for treatment. Exploration revealed that they were being assaulted by their fathers at home. Often, when they were either slapped or pushed by their primitive fathers, they felt frozen and unable to defend themselves, because their enormous dependency needs did not allow them to strike back. They were easily victimized because they feared being expelled from the family. They also feared the loss of their fathers, who had, up to now, defined their "selves" (even though the definition was very negative), and they feared facing the world alone. Their fathers were the obvious "bad objects," since they were physically abusive. However, as in the case of all bad objects, these fathers also displayed some promising and gratifying behaviors. Many of these fathers and sons worked together in the trades, and the identification of these adolescents with a particular trade added some structure to their impoverished identities.

Exploration of the relationship between the sons and their mothers revealed that the mothers were *poorer* objects than the fathers, because they were so inert and uninvolved with their children. Their inertness made them into "nonobjects" unable to meet any developmental needs of their sons. The relief that these young men found from their massive inner tension was to erupt into seemingly unprovoked rages toward authority figures, especially toward the police. This acting-out behavior served to discharge their rage at a symbolically-similar figure while *preserving* the relationship with their needed father. Had they attacked their abusive father directly, they would have been permanently banished from the family. We will see parallels in Walker's description of battering not only in regard to the inhibition of aggression toward the abuser during the first phase of abuse but also in the discharge of rage toward "safe" objects, such as the police, during the battering incident proper.

As the first stage of the battering cycle continues to escalate, the abuser increases the discharge of his now out-of-control abused self:

> His attempts at psychological humiliation become more barbed, his verbal harangues longer and more hostile. Minor battering incidents become more frequent, and the resulting anger lasts for longer periods of time. . . . He hovers around her, barely giving her room to breathe on her own. Tension between the two becomes unbearable. (Walker 1979:59)

This graphic description of the end of the first stage of the battering cycle calls out for some interpretations by Walker. Why do so many men behave like this? She supplies no explanation. As I have noted previously, Walker's model does not allow nonmeasurable internal explanations for the behavior that she observes in these men. Her position is that these men are not acting because of maternal neglect from their childhoods, since she has absolved mothers of all responsibility for their children's development. The victims of abuse are acting equally mysteriously, since the concepts of dependency, complex psychological defenses, impoverished identities, and part-selves cannot be employed in learning-based explanations. Walker's only rationale for the victim's behavior is that she is fearful of physical abuse:

> They cover up for him, make excuses for his rude behavior, and often alienate loved ones who could help them. Some women drive away their parents, sisters, brothers, and often children because they fear they might upset the batterer and then be harmed themselves. (Walker 1979:58)

The reader has an alternate and better explanation for the victim's behavior than Walker presents. The victim of abuse is willing to give up her relationships with her family because her sisters, brothers, and parents are not acting as the (unconsciously chosen) psychological foundation upon which her fragile ego structure rests. As I will show, Walker inadvertently provides evidence for this position. If the victim was truly fearful of the violence, to the exclusion of the intrapsychic factors that I have described, she would leave the abuser *after the very first incident of abuse.* In reality the victim fears that a much greater catastrophe will befall her if she separates from her abuser.

Stage Two—The Acute Battering Incident—Or The Clash of Two Enraged "Abused Selves"

The second phase of the battering cycle described by Walker is called the "acute battering incident." It is characterized by extreme physical violence. Once again, Walker's learning-based model does not permit the use of language that reflects the inner world of either member of the couple who are involved in a battering relationship. If we apply Fairbairn's model to interpret the events so aptly described by Walker, we will see that this stage is characterized by the discharge of the male partner's abused self onto what he now perceives as a totally rejecting object. In effect, it is the full and total discharge of his pent-up frustration and rage at his parents that has been stored in its original state of fury in his abused self. The triggering stimuli for the battering incident might be a need, a want, or a desire that the batterer felt internally but did not express directly to his partner. His infantile vision of the world demands that his adult partner be as attuned to his internal needs as were Winnicott's "good enough mothers," who anticipated their infant's needs prior to the development of language. When his unspoken need is not understood—by his increasingly fearful partner—the batterer's rage erupts into a full-blown fury. After his initial attack the entire reservoir of split off rage in his abused self begins to emerge and once triggered this historical rage becomes uncontrollable.

During this second stage of the battering scenario the victim loses her ability to continue seeing her partner in an unrealistically positive light, as she did in stage one. She can no longer keep her hopeful self in the dominant position when faced with the increasing fury of her violent partner. Her hopeful self is repressed and instantly replaced with her abused self. When her abused self returns to the dominant position, it becomes the mediator of all of her perceptions, and she now sees her partner as an eternally and completely violent monster (which he has become). Once she is dominated by her abused self she is free to retaliate in any way she can, though again the results of the mutual discharge of abused selves *are not remotely comparable.* That is, during the venting of her previously split off rage, the female victim rarely does any physical damage to her abuser, except in those rare cases where she uses a weapon to kill him. This second stage allows the pent up rage in the female victim that was repressed during the mild abuse she suffered in stage one to emerge.

The Psychological Characteristics of the Abusive Male

Let us focus for a moment, before we get to the abuse incident itself, on the general psychological characteristics of the typical batterer. My analysis up to this point has focused on the male batterer's infantile dependency on his partner and his attempt to make up for his developmental deprivation by forcing her to provide him with nurturance that he never received in childhood. I have also described the lack of emotional controls in the batterer that make him volatile and aggressive toward others when he feels deprived. Walker supports these observations in the following quotation, however, she is not able to speculate on the origins of these strong needs in the abusive male. This is because a psychological investigation of his history would implicate the batterer's childhood as the source of his infantile needs. This quote again illustrates Walker's paradoxical ability to describe but not explain the battering scenario.

> Another staple characteristic is the batterer's possessiveness, jealously, and intrusiveness. In order for him to feel secure, he must become overinvolved in the woman's life. In some instances, he may take her to work, to lunch, and bring her home at the end of the working day. . . . Despite this constant surveillance of her every activity, the batterer is still suspicious of his woman's possible relationships with other men and women. (Walker 1979:38)

An object relations analysis of these unanalyzed observations regarding the batterer's extreme need for security is that the batterer is trying to force his new mother substitute to give him all the attention that he missed out on during his developmental history. The batterer acts like a primitive, violent, starving man who has stumbled into a huge restaurant. His ability to control himself is minimal, and his desperation, uncontrolled needs, and enraged emptiness cause him to behave outside the boundaries of normalcy and law.

The paranoia that Walker and others have observed in the batterer is based on his history of abandonment by his parental objects during his childhood. Those barely remembered (or completely repressed) memories of rejection are so painful to him that the batterer does everything in his power to insure that he will not be abandoned again. He uses the independent style, which relies on action, activity, and vigilance, to combat his vulnerability. His paranoia is designed to protect him from the humiliation and potential ego collapse that will occur if his partner leaves him. That is, his paranoid speculations act like an early warning system designed to inform and protect him from the possibility of that abandonment.

Interestingly, many abused women report that the batterer's intense possessiveness was initially attractive to them. This is due to the effects of thousands of painful rejections from their own developmental histories. The future batterer's intense, passionate, and overwhelming interest is welcomed by the developmentally deprived woman, particularly during the initial stages of the relationship. Her self-esteem is buoyed by his intense interest, which feels like a compensation for the hundreds of rejections she experienced at the hands of her her original objects. Naturally, her hopeful self screens out all signs of danger regarding her exciting object's intense, suffocating possessiveness. Her initial feeling of being flattered often turns to horror later on as she realizes that her partner absolutely believes that she is having liaisons behind his back. Over time a victim of abuse recognizes that all her reassurances regarding absolute faithfulness does nothing to reduce the bizarre fears and fantasies in his inner world. This realization—that her partner has lost part of his grip on reality—often serves to *further* activate the victim's bond to her abuser, since she feels she is the only one who knows of his bizarre irrationality. Her misplaced loyalty and sense of responsibility bring her to protect him from being found out. This view of the abusive partner, as being both terrifying and pathetic, has historical precedents in childhood as well. Many abused and neglected children report that they felt enormous attachment to, and responsibility for, the pathetic aspects of their parent, despite the fact that they had been severely mistreated.

Another group of characteristics that are typically found in abusive men are their poor coping skills in the world at large. Often the batterer is fearful of the outside world, which appears to be beyond his control. He is often isolated from his peers, and may have an impoverished interpersonal network. His partner becomes the focus of his need to control his limited and constricted universe. She is also used as a support for his compensatory and grandiose claims of potency, which counteract his feelings of failure in the larger world. His demands that he be regarded as being supremely potent by his partner are backed up by his violence, which is a tangible demonstration of his power.

The final general characteristic of men who batter is their belief in "ultimate" truths and traditional values. The batterer often comes from a background that accepts fundamentalist notions—including the "natural" superiority of men over women. Religion or "the order of the universe" may be used to justify the batterer's dominance over his partner, as if the rules of the heavenly or animal kingdom were somehow relevant to domestic life.

There is a specific event in the histories of male batterers that separates them from men who do not batter women. This is the fact that they saw physical abuse in their home. Once again, I caution the reader against a simplistic learning theory explanation that might postulate that battering is learned in the same way one learns to tie one's shoes. Battering takes place in the context of emotional and physical deprivation. Children who see battering are themselves deprived, needy, angry, and they see the "solution" to the inner hunger displayed by their father, as well as the desperate attachment of their mother to the man who is beating her. Walker quotes some astonishing statistics regarding the effect on the male child of being exposed to battering in the foreword of the Barnett and LaViolette (1993) text. This same quote also demonstrates that Walker has taken a more realistic view of the effects of abuse on the internal structure of the abused woman in the fourteen years since her book was first published:

> Little boys who watch their father abuse their mother are 700 times more likely to use violence in their own homes. If they are abused themselves, that risk factor raises to 1,000 times more. Girls who observe the abuse of their mothers often become victims of spousal abuse as adults. As we learn more about early

abuse, however, it becomes clear that some women use the violence they have learned so well themselves. Those who never learned how to respect another person's boundaries are unable to do so even in therapy. Should their expectations not be met, they strike out just like the batterer taught them. (Barnett and LaViolette: 1993)

The many issues that arise in the therapy of women who have suffered characterological damage because of the effects of this type of early environment will be examined in chapter 6.

An Analysis of the Ego Structure of the Abuser

In previous chapters, victims of abuse have been described as being introjectively insufficient, poorly differentiated from others, and unable to integrate positive and negative images of their objects into a single vision. One of the fundamental positions of this book is that the abuser and the victim of abuse are psychologically similar. As I have noted, the apparent differences between them arise from the contrast between the independent and dependent style rather than from basic differences in their character structures. The psychological similarities are particularly true in terms of the three psychological constructs that were examined in chapter 2.

The most obvious deficiency in the batterer is his lack of internalized good objects. His introjective insufficiency is the motivating force behind his driven, infantile, and overwhelming dependency on his partner. This extreme level of dependency cannot be hidden behind the independent style, and is apparent to even the most casual observer. His infantile demandingness make it clear that he is as internally empty as the woman he is abusing.

The typical batterer also suffers from an inability to remain differentiated from his objects. His poor differentiation from his female partner allows everything that she says or does to enter into his inner world. His hypersensitivity to her every attitude causes him to react to all of her behaviors that are not absolutely congruent with his experience. The only way he can feel comfortable with her is when her positions, opinions, and behaviors are in perfect compliance with his own. Even minor dissension produces powerful feelings of abandonment in him, and the sense that he is completely los-

ing control of his partner. This need for a virtually symbiotic relationship with his partner serves as a psychological replacement for
the early experiences of closeness that were denied him in his own
developmental history. Like an infant, the batterer feels abandoned
the moment he and his object are not feeling the same emotion.

The need to remain in a symbiotic relationship provides an entirely separate source of motivation for the batterer's extreme need to
control his partner when compared to the previously mentioned
motivation for control via physical dominance. The motivation for
physical dominance stemmed from, and was a compensation for, the
batterers feelings of weakness. The motivation for control of his
partner's every feeling state is an attempt on his part to avoid feeling
an intense inner panic when she acts differently from himself. Every
little difference between his inner world and his partner's inner
world signals abandonment and disloyalty to him. One of the often
described (but never explained) consequences of this lack of differentiation is that the batterer believes all of his partner's behaviors
are intended to create a reaction in him. Many batterers justify their
violence toward their partners by claiming that the partner is
responsible for their actions. For instance, a batterer might claim
that his partner is responsible for a particular act of violence on his
part because she "knew" that if she continued to nag him he would
strike out at her. The batterer's ego is unable to modify or attenuate
criticism or demands, and his extreme and violent responses seem
appropriate to him, given the intensity of the experience in his inner
world. The excessive intensity of his innter experience is due to his
lack of a solid ego boundary between himself and his partner. Critical behavior from her pours right into his inner world, and this
immediate, direct, and intense access precludes his diminished ego
from limiting those rageful responses that he may later regret. This
intense form of nondifferentiation was described in chapter 2, both
in the example of Freda and Greta, the intensely undifferentiated
twins, and in the example of Cathy, the secretary whose mother
penetrated every aspect of her life.

Finally, the batterer's underformed ego structure is unable to integrate the two views of his female partner into one whole image. He
sees her as filled with promise when he is in his hopeful self and as
eternally rejecting when he is in his abused self. His inability to integrate comes from exactly the same type of developmental history

experienced by the victim of abuse. As a child, he had to keep his views of his parents unintegrated because a clear (integrated) view of the reality of his childhood would have overwhelmed his ability to cope with the hostility or neglect he was suffering.

The Batterer's Motivation for Abuse of His Partner

If the male partner is so desperately dependent, why does he treat his needed object so badly? Adult logic suggests that you should not kill the golden goose once you have it in your possession. The motivating force for the physical violence that the batterer inflicts on his partner is both sad and simple. The undernurtured male in stage two of the battering scenario acts exactly like the deprived infant would have *liked to act* toward his depriving mother or abusive father—if he could have. However, at the time of his original deprivation he was in the crib, screaming and flailing his arms and legs impotently. Now, this physically mature "adult" is retaliating against his new symbolic mother for failing to supply him with all the attention that he missed out on during his development. His use of the splitting defense does not allow him to see that the "bad" partner he is attacking is the very same woman his hopeful self experiences as the exciting object.

Tragically, the female victim is motivated to cling to the male batterer for similar reasons. She is desperately trying to save herself from the unendurable anxiety attendant to the collapse of her identity, but she relies on the previously mentioned dependent style, which is less active, and uses a strategy of "holding on" to the object no matter what the consequences. Neither individual involved in repeated batterings experienced a history of nurturance or care, and they are both looking for the parenting that they were not given in childhood. Despite the psychological similarities between men and women involved in the battering scenario the consequences for the abuser and the victim are very uneven. The victims of battering are often seriously injured, and may die from their injuries, while the perpetrators of violence often receive mild reprimands or no punishment at all.

Despite his neediness, the male partner viciously attacks his female partner when he is dominated by his abused self. As mentioned, the violent fury of the attack is facilitated by the splitting defense, which cuts the batterer off from all memories of his partner's goodness. He is not only cut off from all good memories of his partner, but he is simultaneously awash in the historical reservoir of pain in his abused self. His partner appears totally frustrating and *deserving* of his rage. The once neglected infant can now strike out at his replacement mother who, he feels, is ignoring his needs. The battering incident itself has been clearly described by Walker:

> In phase two, although he may start out by justifying his behavior to himself, the batterer ends up not understanding what happened. His rage is so great that it blinds his control over his behavior. He starts out wanting to teach the woman a lesson, not intending to inflict any particular injury on her, and stops when he feels she has learned her lesson. By this time, however, she has generally been very severely beaten. (Walker 1976:60)

Once again, Walker supplies us with an excellent description of the battering incident, but offers no reason for this almost "insane" violence on the part of the abuser toward his victim. From Fairbairn's standpoint, this description is an excellent illustration of the primitive power stored in the abused self, as well as the previously described characteristics of low tolerance for frustration and of the acting out defense. After the batterer discharges the pent up rage in his abused self, he loses sight of the hateful feeling that originally triggered the discharge, and cannot remember what provoked him in the first place. The hostile fury of his attack on his partner testifies to the pain of his early memories of neglect and abandonment.

Both Walker's and Barnett and LaViolette's texts describe almost unbelievable examples of physical and sexual abuse. Despite this, the victims remained in relationships with their abusive partners for years. One is simply forced to conclude that the motivation for this attachment to the abusive man is far stronger than the fear of abuse. Walker inadvertently makes an observation that supports this position when she notes that her patients were less anxious when the batterer was with them than when they were living alone.

> Another point we observed relative to depression concerned anxiety levels of battered women. When these women discussed living under the threat and fear of battering there was less anxiety than we expected. *In fact, in many cases it seemed that living with the batterer produced less anxiety than living apart from him.* [My

emphasis.] Why? She often feels that she has the hope of some control if she is with him. Another explanation is that a fear response motivates a search for alternate ways of responding that will avoid or control the threat. Anxiety is, in essence, a call to danger. Physiologically the autonomic nervous system sends out hormones that are designed to cope with immediate stress. Once this stress is under control, anxiety returns to a normal level. Or higher levels of hormones are constantly emitted in order to live under such pervasive stress. This reaction will occur when certain threats are considered uncontrollable. What also happens in this situation is that anxiety does not return to a normal level; rather, it decreases and depression takes over. (Walker 1979:51)

I quoted Walker at length here so that the reader can examine her explanation of why the battered woman is less anxious when her abuser is present than when she is alone. It is not easy to understand, since it includes concepts of physiology, body chemistry, and mastery. Careful reading of it proves to be very difficult, both because of internal inconsistencies and because physical models are mixed with psychological explanations. Walker's analysis of the reasons behind the battered woman's lowered anxiety when her abusing partner is with her is unsatisfactory because her model excludes discussion of the internal motivating factors that orchestrate the complex interpersonal transactions constituting the typical battering scenario.

The Fairbairnian explanation for this observation comes to a more reasonable conclusion: that the victim of abuse is less fearful when the batterer is present, *despite the fact that she may suffer more abuse*, because she needs him to stabilize her damaged sense of self. Conversely, the victim is more anxious when she is alone because she risks the collapse of her ego. This is the identical observation that Fairbairn made sixty years ago. His abused children were more anxious in the foundling home than when they were at home, despite the fact that they risked further injury at home. The victim's increased comfort when the batterer is present speaks of her need for an object that serves to keep her identity intact. It is both the male abuser's pseudo strength and the victim's hope for the continuation of the relationship with him that keeps her ego from collapse. Once again the physical abuse is not the key issue but rather the absolute dependency that the victim has on her needed partner. Without his presence, her weak inner structure, her introjective insufficiency, her lack of identity, and her fear of the world all threaten to annihilate her. Walker's analysis of the battering scenario is compromised because she cannot address the inner world of either the batterer or the victim.

The most interesting aspect of the battering incident described by Walker, and the one that gives her interpretation of events its greatest test, is the high probability that the abused woman will attack the police when they come to her aid. This common reaction of battered women is another politically difficult reality to explain:

> Police also complain of being attacked by the women themselves if they attempt to intervene during a phase two incident. They become understandably indignant when the very person they set out to help turns on them. They interpret her behavior as complicity with her husband's violence. What they fail to understand is that the battered woman knows that when the police leave she will be left alone with the batterer again, and she is terrified of being further abused. When she attacks the police she is trying to demonstrate her loyalty to her batterer, hoping to avert further beating. (Walker 1979:64–65)

By excluding all that we know about the interior world of both the abuser and the victim Walker is unable to come to an accurate conclusion regarding the victim's motivation for her attack on the police. In fact, the conclusion that Walker reaches, that the victim fears being left alone with the batterer—flies in the face of her own observations. If the battered woman is primarily terrified of violence, why does she remain in the relationship year after year? Moreover, why is she less anxious when she is with the abuser than when she is alone? The prior example of the teen-aged boys who were fearful of retaliating against their needed but abusive fathers but thought nothing of spitting in a policeman's face, serves as an exact analogy to this situation. Fear of beating is not the basic motivation of the battered woman (or of the teen-aged boy, for that matter), rather it is the fear in the victim of the loss of her desperately needed object and the resulting collapse of her sense of self.

Learning theory, when applied properly to this situation, would interpret that there is a positive reinforcer present that is greater than the pain from the negative reinforcement (the physical abuse). That is, a strong reinforcer is able to overcome a strong punishment, as long as the reinforcer is more positive than the punishment is negative. In terms of the battering scenario, it is less punishing for the borderline woman to tolerate the beatings than it is to face the possibility of the collapse of her understructured ego.

When we look at the same observations using Fairbairn's model we can see two related motivations for the attack on the police: 1. the victim (like the teen-aged youth) cannot control the discharge of rage from her abused self, which is dominant during the abuse phase, however, she cannot destroy her abuser either, because of her extreme dependency needs on him; and 2. the police have the power to take her abuser away, and she will be faced with the possible collapse of her ego structure.

When the police arrive the battered woman is operating out of her abused self, and she sees all objects as "bad." No remnant of her hopeful self, which was dominant during the first phase of the battering scenario, exists. The abused self is filled with rage and hate, and the police serve as a "safe" target for the discharge of her rage, particularly when compared to the desperately needed spouse she cannot attack with the same impunity. Aggression directed toward the police will not affect her dependency relationship with her partner. This is the reason the abused teenager would rather spit in a policeman's face than defend himself against his father's physical abuse.

Moreover, the battered woman attacks the police because they threaten to end the battered woman's dependency relationship on her abuser. If the police take the victim's violent partner away to jail, her sense of self might collapse, which is the worst fate that she can imagine. Therefore she perceives the police as a threat to her dependency relationship, and attacks. Thus the violence and brutality she endures at the hands of her partner is less important to her than the danger posed by the loss of her dependency relationship on him.

This complex, intrapsychic view of the observable data poses difficult problems for advocates of battered women who want the victim of abuse to be seen as a totally passive, nonparticipating outsider who has just happened to find an abusive man. Walker's hypothesis, that the victim's attack on the police is motivated by terror of being left alone with the batterer after the police leave, is an absolutely incorrect conclusion. The victim is, in fact, terrified that she will be left alone *without* the batterer, and Walker's earlier observation that the victim is more anxious when alone than with her abuser supports this view.

Frustrated Dependency and Suicide-Homicide

The ultimate aspect of infantile dependency in male batterers can be seen in those cases where the female victim manages to leave the relationship. Walker reports that almost 10 percent of the batterers in her study killed themselves after their female partners left. Once again, Walker's observations are not followed by any interpretation of the data. In effect, these men are so infantile and dependent that their sense of self collapses after their abused (yet desperately needed) object flees. The abuser may appear on the surface to be far more intact than his victim, because he uses the independent pattern, which gives him a superficial aura of strength. However, once he has lost his victim the the many similarities between battered women and the men that abuse them emerge. The abuser's ego structure and identity is, as I have mentioned, as weak as that of his victim. Sadly, many batterers kill not only themselves, but their partner as well, when the victim begins to withdraw from the relationship.

Once again I turn to the June 17, 1992, issue of the *Journal of the American Medical Association* for its perspective on this type of crime. Approximately one thousand to fifteen hundred people are killed in this country every year in these double crimes, with half to three quarters of the murders motivated by what Marzuk, Tardiff, and Hirsch called "amorous jealousy":

> Typically, a male between the age of 18 and 60 years develops suspicions or knowledge of his girlfriend's or wife's infidelity, becomes enraged, and both murders her and commits suicide. . . . Most often there has been a chronically chaotic relationship fraught with jealous suspicions, verbal abuse, and sub-lethal physical violence. The triggering event is often the female's rejection of her lover and her immediate threat of withdrawal or estrangement.
> (Marzuk, Tardiff, and Hirsch 1992:3,180)

This quote again reinforces the perspective that the infantile aspect of these men emerges when they face the threat of abandonment. I was asked to comment on this phenomenon by a local television station a number of years ago. Vermont saw a series of killings that involved couples having long histories of violence. Of particular interest was the case of a batterer who had been legally restrained from seeing his desperately needed girlfriend-victim. This couple had a long and violent history with each other, and the female partner had finally begun to withdraw from the relationship. The batterer returned to her home, kidnapped her, and deliberately ran his car into a tree at high speed, killing them both instantly. The press came to me because they could not understand why this "adult" man would kill himself, although they did "understand" why *he* killed *her*. It is hard for the general public to conceptualize adult-looking human beings who function at the emotional level of infants. Once this concept is grasped, this common type of murder-suicide scenario is easily understood. In effect, this infant/man had been abandoned by his replacement mother. This abandonment provoked the reemergence of all the childhood rage stored in his abused self. In his rage his infantile psyche directed his adult body to destroy his abandoning "all bad" object. Once he was committed to this course of action, his own life was over as well, for without his partner his ego was sure to collapse. The collapse of the abuser's ego and sense of self is equivalent to psychological death. His physical life cannot continue, since he is not be able to exist alone, and so his suicide is easily understood.

The Third Stage: The Reemergence of Two Hopeful Selves

The third phase of the battering scenario begins after the primitive rage from the abused self of the batterer is discharged. Walker calls this phase "kindness and contrite loving behavior," and here the reader can see the splitting defense in its most blatant form. Walker describes the male batterer's shift back to his hopeful self after his abused self is fully discharged by the violence:

> The third phase follows immediately on the second and brings with it an unusual period of calm. The tension built up in phase one and released in phase two is gone. In this phase, the batterer constantly behaves in a charming and loving manner. He begs her forgiveness and promises her that he will never do it again.
> (Walker 1979:65)

The object relations explanation of the abuser's sudden shift from one part self to the other begins with the same observation made by

Walker, that the discharge of his abused self leaves him in a relatively neutral state. He is no longer pressured by unendurable tension. The discharge of aggression deflates his abused self, and this paves the way for his hopeful self to return to dominance. The discharge of the abused self does not stimulate the hopeful self to return, rather, it leaves him in a state of low tension, which reduces the resistance to the return of the split off hopeful self. The specific stimulus that activates the return of the hopeful self after the battering incident is the abuser's realistic fear that he may lose his partner because of his brutality toward her. The thought that she may leave him reactivates his awareness of how much he needs her. His recognition of his need shifts his perception away from the view of her as a rejecting object and back to the opposite view of her as an exciting object. He suddenly sees her as containing the promise of future love for him. This stimulates the hopeful self to return to the dominant position in his inner world, which was left "open" by the discharge of his abused self.

The moment the abuser splits back into his hopeful self he sets out to manipulate his victim to split back into her hopeful self. He must work quickly because he is faced with the possibility that she will remain in her abused self long enough to make the decision to leave him. The abuser will try to get her to see him as as an exciting object once again, thus provoking the return of her hopeful self. If she has sought help, he must swiftly counter the efforts of the professionals who will likely urge her to remain separate from him. The abuser's frenetic efforts to "recapture" his partner are described by Walker, although she offers absolutely no psychological explanation for this *stunning* reversal on the part of the abuser:

> These women were thoroughly convinced of their desire to stop being victims, until the batterer arrived. I always knew when a woman's husband had made contact with her by the profusion of flowers, candy, cards and other gifts in her hospital room. By the second day, the telephone calls and visits intensified, as did his pleas to be forgiven and promises never to do it again. He usually engaged others in his fierce battle to hold on to her. His mother, father, sisters, brothers, aunts, uncles, friends, and anyone else he could commandeer would call and plead his case to her.
>
> (Walker 1979:66)

This quote illustrates how aware the batterer is of his partner's hopeful self. His exaggerated efforts to appear to be loving are designed to restimulate hope in his partner's split off hopeful self. On the surface the batterer appears to be making a totally manipulative play on his partner's weak ego and lack of will. Most batters appear sly and outright evil during this stage of the battering scenario as they work furiously to reactivate the hopeful self in their partners psyche. It must be kept in mind that the batterer also uses the splitting defense, and his abused self is no longer available to his consciousness. He cannot remember the hate, rage, and murderousness that he discharged toward his partner because his abused self is now repressed. Therefore much of his behavior is less overtly manipulative than it appears to be. Walker also notes, but does not explain, the sincerity of the batterer now that his abused self is safely repressed: "The batterer truly believes he will never again hurt the woman he loves; he believes he can control himself from now on" (Walker 1979:65). The enormous and uncanny power of the splitting defense to isolate a set of memories from the abuser's awareness explains his sincerity.

It is not surprising that these tactics work wonders on the battered woman. Her own history with unreliable parents, who repeatedly rejected her and then reversed their position and accepted her, created an inner structure that responds to strong displays of hopeful behavior from her (mostly) rejecting partner. This time it is her abuser instead of her parents who reverses position. Her abusing partner does most of the work for her, work that she used to do by herself in her childhood. As a child she preserved her relationship with her rejecting parents with exaggerated fantasies of love that were held in her hopeful self. Now, her partner transforms himself into an exciting object and works assiduously to reactivate her split off hopeful self. Her partner begs for forgiveness, unlike her parents who she wished would ask for forgiveness, but never did. Her partner's exaggerated behaviors are almost a dream-come-true for the abused woman, and she typically has little ability to resist the pull of her reinstated hopeful self. The entire abuse/reunion cycle is dependent on the presence of splitting *in both partners*. It returns to the well-worn psychological mechanisms that were developed in both members of the battering dyad during their childhoods. The abuser's contrite and loving behavior gradually activates the hopeful self in the victim, as described by Walker:

> The battered woman wants to believe that she will no longer have to suffer abuse. The batterer's reasonableness supports her belief that he really can change, as does his loving behavior during this phase. She convinces herself that he can do what he says he wants to do. It is during this phase that the woman gets a glimpse of her original dream of how wonderful he is. . . . The battered woman chooses to believe that the behavior she sees during phase three signifies what her man is really like. She identifies the good man with the man she loves. He is now everything she ever wanted in a man. (Walker 1979:67–68)

Once again, Walker has absolutely no psychological explanation in her model for this striking, stunning, almost unbelievable reversal on the part of the victim. She presents this reversal as if it is based on a moment of faulty logic. In reality, this reversal is a major psychological event. As she notes, it often takes place in the *hospital room* just days after the woman has been severely beaten! It is as dramatic as the emergence of a second personality in an individual afflicted with multiple personality disorder. The lack of any psychological explanation for this shift by Walker demonstrates the dilemma of the learning theorist faced with the problem of explaining human behavior without knowing about the splitting defense and without understanding the inner world of the victim.

The reader, again, has a more potent and cohesive explanation for this shift than the does Walker. The sudden reversal of perceptions in the victim is based on the repression of the formerly dominant abused self, which is then replaced by the newly unrepressed hopeful self. The artful manipulations of the batterer, which begin almost immediately after physical violence, changes the victim's perception of him from a rejecting object back to an exciting object. Once the abuser is seen by the victim as containing potential love, the hopeful self becomes the dominant part-ego. This switch can only happen if the female partner has the splitting defense well established in her inner world.

This shift from one sense of self to the other poses an enormous problem for all the helping professions, particularly those who are not aware of the inner structure and dynamics of the human psyche: "Helpers of battered women become exasperated at this point, since the women will usually drop charges, back down on separation or divorce, and generally try to patch things up until the next acute incident" (Walker 1979:68).

Can you imagine the well-intentioned worker, unaware of the fundamental structural defenses in battered women, who is trying to work with this population? What could possibly be more frustrating than for the rescue-oriented worker to see the battered woman suddenly split from the pain-laden abused self back to the naive, unrealistic, hopeful self. At this point the battered woman will most often return home with the contrite abuser. The worker knows that another episode of abuse is lurking around the corner, but the victim who uses the splitting defense cannot remember the material repressed in her abused self.

The splitting off of the abused selves in both partners places them on a temporary honeymoon, but it also prepares the ground for another first phase build-up of tension. Walker notes that many of the 120 women she studied had become skillful at prolonging the phase three loving behavior in their partners. However, four of the women from her sample who had been repeatedly battered killed their male partners when phase one battering resumed. These cases probably occurred, again using Fairbairn's perspective, because the female partner was not able to sustain her hopeful self during the first phase as she had in the past. These four women probably had their abused self emerge before they were exhausted by the abuse. The abused self of the battering victim contains the rage from her childhood plus the rage from her recent abuses, and it is powerful enough in many cases to destroy the batterer.

The Learning Theory Explanation of the Attachment of the Victim to the Batterer

Walker's explanatory model for the battering cycle is an area of learning theory that is called "learned helplessness." She sees learning theory as a positive alternative to prior attempts to explain the battering syndrome by theorists who used concepts like "intrapsychic conflict" that she claims have not worked out:

> Prior research on family violence has tended to be clinically oriented and to focus on the pathology of the individuals involved,

primarily the intrapsychic conflicts of the man and the woman. The research that I have been conducting since 1975 suggests this approach is inadequate for understanding the battered woman problem. (Walker 1979:43)

Walker's book began the trend in the field of using learning theory and, specifically, the concept of "learned helplessness" to explain the dynamics of battering. This trend has continued to the present, and the most recent text I have seen on battering, Barnett and LaViolette's *It Could Happen To Anyone* (1993), sits in this theoretical camp as well. This model fits nicely with the politically based goal of eliminating all possibility that the victim has any conscious or unconscious role in the battering scenario by focusing on the consequences of beating on the victim's behavior. It denies that the victim has a deep and abiding attachment to the abuser, and instead assumes that she is with him because she is too damaged by the abuse to escape. Barnett's and LaViolett's title announces their position, which is completely incorrect in the light of the model that I have described. In fact battering, when it is defined by multiple instances of abuse, cannot happen to just anyone. It can only happen when the victim has had a history that severely compromised her ego structure.

Walker's explanatory model is based on animal research in which dogs in cages were given electrical shocks. The shocks came on a variable interval schedule, which simply means that they came after randomized periods of time, which were impossible for the dogs to predict. The shocks were also completely independent of the dogs' behavior. Over a short period of time the dogs learned that they could do nothing to prevent or escape from the shocks. They became passive and inert, and later attempts to teach the dogs how to escape the shocks were nearly impossible. Walker then draws an analogy between the dogs' belief (which were a consequence of the experiment) that nothing they did could, or would, make a difference with the beliefs and behaviors of the abused women:

> Repeated batterings, like electrical shocks, diminish the woman's motivation to respond. She becomes passive. Secondly, her cognitive ability to perceive success is changed. She does not believe her response will result in a favorable outcome, whether or not it might. (Walker 1979:50)

Once again, I must point out that Walker has missed the key issue, which is that the victim of battering *does not want to flee the batterer*, just like Fairbairn's children did not want to be separated from their abusive parents. Walker manages to ignore or not explain the stunning reversals in both the abuser and victim, while those interpretations she does make regarding the victim's decreased anxiety when her batterer is present, and her explanation for the victim's attack on the police, are confusing and inadequate when compared to the alternative analysis derived from Fairbairn's work.

The learned helplessness that Walker cites as the key to understanding the behavior of the victim is not a consequence of the battering but rather the consequence of the victim's developmental history. Walker cannot accept this because it suggests that the victim has character problems, and this opens the possibility of another round of blaming the victim. In fact, my discussion has demonstrated that the battered woman has been severely shortchanged twice in her life, and that there is something fundamentally wrong with a culture that allows this cycle of childhood deprivation/abuse followed by adulthood abuse to continue. The abused woman is helpless in the same way that a child is helpless. These women are helpless before they ever met the batterer, because their own family of origin did not support them enough for them to develop the ego structure and identity that is essential for adulthood. Now that the issue of the battering cycle is understood, it is time to look at an approach to repairing the battered woman.

Summary

This chapter has focused on the actual battering scenario, and compared the analysis originating from Fairbairn's object relations theory to the analysis offered by Lenore Walker using learning theory to explain the same observations. The delicate political issue of the battered woman's unconscious attraction to men who end up as abusers was examined in the light of the victim's history with her unreliable parents, which created two separate part-selves in her inner world. These two selves, the abused self and the hopeful self, relate to, and resonate with, high intensity rejecting behaviors followed by promising behaviors from characterologically disordered men. The hopeful self in the victim is attracted to the promise and fantasy of love from her partner, and her abused self is attracted to rejecting behaviors on the part of her partner. The attraction of the abused self to rejecting aspects of men is a reversal of the normal human pattern of fleeing from those who are unreliable and rejecting. The borderline woman feels understood by men who "speak" to these separate selves in her, and, conversely, she is intimidated by normal men who do not have any knowledge of, or tolerance for, her part-selves.

The analytic concept that defines the reenactment of childhood patterns in adult relationships is called repetition compulsion, and it was another one of Freud's original contributions to the field. He was so impressed with its power that he modified his central concept of the pleasure principle by hypothesizing a death instinct that opposed his libidinal instincts. Freud's explanation for the "compulsion to repeat" was that the individual was trying to master the early trauma that overwhelmed him as a child. This explanation seems to be partly correct, although it misses the core issue that the adult is recreating the same form of emotional attachment that he experienced as a child. The second model of repetition compulsion is Fairbairn's, and it holds that the adult is attracted to the same mix of antithetical emotions that she experienced in childhood, including intense closeness, rejection, hate, and longing for love. These feelings change suddenly, and follow one another in a bewildering and unpredictable pattern. The six factors that work together to bond the abused woman to her partner include:

1. the child's inability to protect herself from abuse, which results in a malformed ego structure and impoverished identity
2. the child's (and immature adult's) intense focus on one, and only one, person for gratification of dependency needs
3. the internal pressure from unmet needs for nurturance that were never gratified in childhood and erupt in adulthood
4. the extreme dependency on others due to either a) the lack of a clear identity, which requires the partner's pseudo strength to keep that identity from collapse for those individuals using the dependent pattern, or b) the inability to self-soothe, which is the result of introjective insufficiency most common in the independent pattern character disorders
5. the twin defenses, splitting and the moral defense against bad objects, that hide the "badness" of the abuser from his victim

6. the previously mentioned attraction of the victim's part-selves to the pattern of alternating rejecting and loving behaviors typical of abusers

The battering cycle, called the "cycle theory of violence" in Walker's book *The Battered Woman*, was then analyzed using Fairbairn's object relations theory. The first stage of the battering cycle occurs when the infantile abuser feels that his needs are not being met or when he uses his partner as an easy target for rage that may have developed from frustrations outside the relationship. During this stage the batterer is dominated by his abused self, and he sees his partner as a rejecting object. The female victim attempts to remain in her hopeful self, and uses the splitting defense and the moral defense to hide from the reality of the abuser's "badness." The male partner is extremely dependent on his victim, as shown by his possessiveness and jealousy. He behaves like an empty, greedy, tyrannical infant in an adult body, who attempts to squeeze the maximum quantity of "nurturance" from his symbolic mother. The male abuser physically attacks his desperately needed partner because of his enormous reservoir of unmet needs, which are beyond anyone's ability to satisfy, and the reservoir of rage at his original parents for their deprivation of him.

The battering incident is acted out by the two abused selves that are dominant in both partners. The abuser feels that he is justified because of his inner emptiness, and the victim's abused self is based on her historical deprivation coupled with the now expressed rage from the current incident and past incidents of battering. It is during the second stage of the battering incident that the police may be called to intervene, and there is a good chance that the battered woman will attack those who have been sent to rescue her. The explanation for this puzzling behavior is based on the massive dependency of the victim on her batterer. Her ego may collapse if she looses her desperately needed object when the police take him away, and she does her best to protect him from this fate. Interestingly, Walker also notes that the victim of abuse, who she claims is terrified of further abuse, is less anxious when her abuser is living with her than when she is alone. This was exactly the case with Fairbairn's abused children in Scotland.

The third stage of the battering scenario occurs when the abuser feels that all the rage in his abused self is discharged, and his hopeful self becomes the dominant ego state. He fears the loss of his exciting object, who, he now feels, contains the hope of future love for him. He exaggerates his loving behavior toward his perhaps hospitalized partner, and his performance is often enough to cause her to split back into her hopeful self and repress her abused self. This is an almost unbelievable shift, as the victim might still be covered with physical reminders of the abuse. Despite this, the powerful psychological defense of splitting takes over and blots out the painful reality and replaces it with the fantasies lodged in her hopeful self.

CHAPTER SIX

An Object
Relations Approach
to the Psychotherapy
of the Battered Woman

In my previous book, *Treatment of the Borderline Patient: Apply ing Fairbairn's Object Relations Theory in the Clinical Setting*, I described in detail treatment procedures that are effective in repairing the structural damage to the personality that is found in people with borderline disorders. My goal in this chapter is limited to outlining the areas of ego functioning that are typically in need of repair in victims of physical abuse. Not surprisingly, I will again refer to the three basic ego functions of differentiation, integration, and introjection. Unlike the discussion in chapter 2, I am going to start with introjection, because the two other processes cannot begin until memories of support from the therapeutic relationship are taken into the internal world of the abused woman.

Before I get to that discussion it must be mentioned that I have found that the treatment of victims of abuse is more practical and effective than the treatment of the typical male abuser. There are a number of reasons for this, all of which come up in my previous discussion of the characteristics of the abuser. The first difficulty that one faces when treating the male abuser is based on his use of the independent style. The abuser insists in seeing himself as dominant and in control. He cannot admit to any feelings of dependency, and will avoid placing himself in a position of obvious dependence on others who are more powerful than himself as he is haunted by memories of abuse from his childhood. His dependency needs have been (up to this time) focused on his partner, whom he could control completely. He will ferociously resist the demand for compliance that is required of all patients, as well as the role of the child looking for approval from a (potentially aggressive) parentlike therapist. Typically, the abuser has constructed a closed and artificial universe where he has made and enforced all the rules. The therapy situation places him in a foreign interpersonal world in which he is subject to a whole new set of rules that bring his every attitude into question. It is frightening and enraging for him to be questioned about his behaviors or to place himself under the control of anyone. One of the most common pathways that leads the abuser to therapy is through a court order as a condition of his release. The levels of suppressed rage that develop in the abuser from this situation cannot be underestimated and this rage often destroys the possibility of the development of a therapeutic alliance. Many men resist the therapeutic endeavor by attempting to act in a charming and innocent manner in the hope of deceiving the individual responsible for treatment. In contrast, female victims of abuse are comfortable with their feelings of dependency. They do not feel demeaned when they are in a dependent relationship, and they are used to seeking strength in others. Thus the therapeutic relationship fits their needs and does not threaten them.

The second difficulty in treating male abusers stems from the reality that some percentage of abusers (which I will not venture to estimate) are psychopathic personality disorders. This is the reciprocal of my earlier point that most female victims of abuse are borderline types but some are even more disturbed than the typical borderline. Briefly, a psychopath is an amplified narcissist. Individuals with this major personality disorder are far more primitive, empty, deceptive, revenge driven, and dangerous than are narcissistic personality disorders. Do not assume that all psychopaths are in jail or are easy to identify. On the contrary, they are often exceedingly adept at role playing, and can imitate a "normal" person so well that others who meet them after a violent assault on their partner simply cannot believe they are capable of the damage that they have committed. This ability to role-play is a consequence of an extreme lack of identity. Without a real self, the psychopath has no permanent personality that has to be "pushed aside" when taking on a new role. Tragically, the psychopath's acting ability is a key asset in his ability to win back the partner that he has just beaten. He is able to make grand gestures of "love" that are alluring to the hopeful self operative in his victim. In addition to this almost complete inner emptiness there is a deep and abiding rage, vast and unquenchable needs, and a hostile desire for vengeance. The psychopathic abuser who is forced to be a "patient" will show superficial compliance with the treatment while plotting the murder of his traitorous partner, the dismemberment of the therapist, and the annihilation of the judge who sentenced him. Not all abusers are this disturbed, however, the combination of resistance to treatment from average abusers due to their use of the independent style and the added problems of dealing with psychopathic abusers makes treatment of this population a daunting prospect. In general, the goal of my treatment with abused women is to repair their damaged ego structure to the point that they have no interest *whatsoever* in the type of man who overplays love and follows soon afterward with physical abuse.

Introjection of the Therapist—The Foundation of Change

In chapter 2 I noted the close relationship between introjection and differentiation. The child who has supportive parent(s) is able to build up a large collection of positive memories that then allow her to explore the world without fear. The more internal support she has, the more readily she is able to differentiate from her mother. The same principle holds true in reverse for the battered woman. She is unable to differentiate from her abusive partner because she does not have enough positive introjects to hold her ego structure together in the absence of her object.

Simply stated, it is *impossible* for the abused woman to separate from her needed object until she has internalized many ego-structuring memories of support from the therapeutic relationship. Therefore introjection is the first goal of the therapeutic program, not differentiation. Naturally, the treatment plan that I am outlining is based on outpatient treatment for the abused woman. This plan assumes that the patient is not in extreme danger. When the patient is in mortal danger, other approaches—the most common being to remove the victim, and children, from her home and into a battered women's shelter, is the best (and often only) course of action. This affords protection from more abuse, which in many cases is essential. However, the move often forces an abused woman to behave in ways for which she is not psychologically prepared. That is, she may be very reluctant to leave her abuser, and will be faced with the very difficult task of maintaining her sense of self without him. The long-term goal of the outpatient treatment plan that I am describing is to strengthen the victim's ego gradually so that she is able to resist the temptation to return to her abuser after she leaves the supportive therapeutic environment.

The great difficulty in working with the battered woman lies in the simple fact that the victim depends on the abuser for her psychological life. In Fairbairn's terms, she is stubbornly attached to her bad object because, paradoxically, he is the only one she trusts. To the outsider, the abuser often appears to be an awful choice of a partner. However, as I have described, his power over his victim is the result of his repeated promise to love her in the future. In order for outpatient therapy to be successful, the abused woman has to give up her attachments to her abuser and shift her massive dependency needs onto the relationship with her "good object" therapist. Fairbairn understood that the cure for patients who suffered from attachments to bad objects was for the therapist to behave as an "unwontonly good object." The patient's positive attachment to the therapist will gradually displace her attachment to exciting but frustrating objects. This approach places a great burden on the therapist because it allows and encourages the patient to focus all of her enormous dependency needs on him or her. This reality scares many mental health professionals, who are uncomfortable when faced with extreme levels of patient dependency needs and tend to shy away from treating this difficult population.

This therapeutic approach does not mean that the therapist capitulates to the patient's reservoir of unmet needs by indulging her with extended sessions, long phone conversations, or "regressing" the patient to experience the symbiotic closeness she (and perhaps the therapist as well) missed out on as a child. Rather, the therapist has to act in a reliable and predictable manner so that the abused woman can get used to counting on support from another human being. The therapist has to provide these patients with the equivalent of the soothing memories that the air force photographer called upon when he was drowning in hot gasoline. How does this process happen? In truth, it happens slowly over time, like grains of sand falling in an hourglass. Each small positive introject weighs little individually. However, when the critical mass is achieved, the glass suddenly turns upside down. The therapist's absolute reliability, her interest in the patient, her integrity, and honesty offer the patient new experiences of support that ultimately form a new mass of positive introjects. Because of the gradual nature of the introjection process, very little appears to happen at the outset of therapy as there are too few positive introjects to alter the patient's normal coping strategies.

Four Major Obstacles to the Introjection of the Therapist

Despite the fact that introjection is the key process necessary to repair the battered woman, there are a number of formidable obstacles to block this process. These obstacles are called resistances, and include patient expectations, fears, and beliefs that are the result of the deprived histories from which these women emerged. One or more of these resistances can stop all therapeutic progress and leave the abused woman in her damaged state without hope of repair. The reader who has never worked with this population might assume that the abused woman is a compliant and willing patient. *Nothing* could be further from the truth. As I have noted, the abused woman is not threatened by the therapeutic situation, however, once involved, her resistances to change will emerge. I will describe four major areas of resistance that can crop up in the psychotherapy of the battered woman. Despite the fact that they are discussed separately, more than one problem can emerge in the work with any given patient.

The Victim's Suspicion of the Therapist's "Goodness"

The first impediment to the patient's acceptance and internalization of the therapist's efforts is her suspicion of the therapist's motivation. The most potent source of "cumulative trauma" experienced by neglected children at the hands of their parents is the unreliability of the normal routines of daily life. They are never sure if one parent or the other is going to be home, or is going to explode into a rage, or if even the most elemental of caretaking events can be counted upon. The child burdened by this type of history learns very quickly to take up the slack: by anticipating her parents' moods or by learning to care for herself. No matter how adept the child becomes at fending for herself, she will be wary of anyone who offers her parentlike help, holding the firm belief that she will be used once again in the therapeutic relationship as she was in the parent-child relationship. Thus, when a patient with this type of history enters into a therapeutic relationship, she expects the worst, and the therapist's job is to reverse this expectation.

Most often battered women begin therapy in a confused, fearful, and wary state. The therapist's role is to calmly interpret the patient's fears in terms of her theoretical model and experience. The therapist is offering herself to the patient as an auxiliary ego, and applies her thought processes, her strategies, and her model to the patient's problems. Despite this humane and genuine offer by the therapist, the abused patient is so convinced that all intimate object relationships are exploitative and temporary that she is unwilling to believe anyone can offer her real help. She will probe the therapist's implied goodwill toward her by testing the strength of the *framework*. This is the term most often used to describe the conditions under which therapy occurs (Langs 1973a, b), and it refers to the therapist's style—the hours, fees, privacy, and regularity of the clinical interviews. For instance, the wary patient may predict that the therapist will not hold to his or her offer to help, either because the patient's problems are boring or because the patient is not important enough for the therapist to be concerned with. The patient will be hypersensitive and vigilant to the therapist's every move, and if she or he displays a momentary lapse in attention the patient will victoriously point out that the therapist is indeed bored, or uninterested. If the therapy dyad consists of a female patient and a male therapist, and the patient's family of origin had poor boundaries, she might suggest they meet outside of the office in a social situation so that they can "get to know each other better." In this manner the patient offers to involve herself in a therapeutic corruption of the framework in order to see if the therapist is as willing to violate the rules as were her own parents. These patients fear that the therapist is untrustworthy while at the same time they hope that he or she is not. Despite their hope, when the therapist proves reliable many patients will still not accept the therapist's reliability as real.

The Negative Therapeutic Reaction

A second and more serious possibility for difficulties in the internalization of the therapist's effort to help is called the *negative therapeutic reaction* (Seinfeld 1990, Celani 1993). The negative therapeutic reaction is defined as the deterioration of the patient despite appropriate and timely interventions by the therapist. This occurs in two separate ways. The most common pattern is the result of a patient's severe mistreatment in childhood having left such indelible marks on her that she projects memories of her past abuser onto the therapist. She then reacts to him or her *as if* the therapist is equivalent to the original rejecting object, and responds with hate and suspicion from her abused self. This "mistake" by the patient is called *transference*, and it is arguably Freud's greatest clinical discovery. The patient transfers the powerful negative feelings that she developed in her relationships with her parents onto the therapist, and then behaves as if her therapist is identical to her original objects.

The second form of the negative therapeutic reaction originates in the patient's introjection of her parents' hostile attitudes, which were originally directed toward her. This is a well-known phenomenon, and has been observed by an individual as far removed from psychology as Sir Richard Burton, the English linguist and translator. He is famous for the quote "The goal of every slave is not freedom, but a slave of his own." From his observation of cultures with slavery Burton understood that once an individual is involved in a master/slave relationship he is forever locked into one or the other of these two roles. That is, both the slave and the master cannot imagine a relationship that does not include domination or subjugation. In terms of the negative therapeutic reaction, the patient attempts to dominate his therapist with criticism and rejection in exactly the same manner in which he was enslaved as a child. Many patients, including the previously mentioned man who was chased around the lawn by his enraged father, report that later in life they find themselves behaving just like those parts of their parents they hated most. In terms of the internal components this form of the negative therapeutic reaction occurs when the patient reenacts the role of the internalized rejecting object in relation to the therapist. The internalized rejecting object is the collection of memories of the parent(s) when they attacked, rejected, or demeaned the child. The patient behaves as hatefully and as critically toward the therapist as her parents behaved toward her in childhood.

This style of negative therapeutic reaction differs markedly from the first type in that the prior negative transference was based on the patient's mistaken belief that she was in the presence of a dangerous abuser. Under those conditions, her fearful, abused self emerged to combat what she misperceived to be an abuser. This second form occurs when the patient acts as the protagonist and actively attacks and attempts to victimize the therapist. When this happens the therapist is forced into exactly the same position in which the patient was once caught. The patient will attack the therapist for being stupid, insensitive to her needs, or otherwise demean the therapist's best efforts. In response to the patient's attack the therapist might develop a "mini" abused self and feel as if he or she is unable to do anything correctly.

In either case, these tenacious, long-term, hostile transferences become classified as negative therapeutic reactions when they go on for month after month, and disrupt or destroy the therapeutic relationship.

The Out of Contact Patient

A third form of resistance that may prevent the patient from internalizing the therapist occurs when the patient enters therapy in the "out of contact stage" (Searles 1965, Seinfeld 1990, Celani 1993). This condition is very different from the previously described negative therapeutic reaction. Basically, the patient who enters therapy in the out of contact stage is one who has so few expectations of support due to her past history that she enters the consulting room in a near daze, and may not even be able to process the words said by the therapist. These patients often had so little parental support as children that they cannot conceive of anyone helping them in any way. Patients who begin therapy in the out of contact stage will wonder aloud why they are in the consulting room, ask if they should return, or become disturbed by the therapist's concern for them. This last factor is the result of such severe neglect that they are frightened at the prospect of someone else becoming affected by their distress. Another indication that the patient is in the out of contact stage is when she reports that she regularly forgets the entire interactional content of each session the moment she leaves the office. The obvious task for the therapist who is faced with this type of patient is to penetrate her awareness with the reality that he or she is there to assist with her problems in life.

The Patient's Insistence on Her Own Explanation for Her Plight

The fourth problem area that interferes with the patient's willingness to internalize the therapist's efforts to help is often the most difficult form of resistance to surmount. Basically, it involves the "debate" between the therapist and the patient as to why she is having so much trouble in her life. Each patient has a "model" of her own as to why she is in a battering relationship, and she will insist that her model is correct while simultaneously rejecting the therapist's position. Many use the previously described moral defense to rationalize why they are being abused. Often the patient has a whole series of separate and contradictory explanations for her plight. This is not at all surprising, since the patient has had to explain repeatedly both to herself and to her friends why she has remained in a destructive, perhaps life-threatening relationship. It is akin to explaining why you continue to hit yourself on the head with a hammer. The explanation must be powerful enough to convince both the abused woman and her friends that her relationship is, at the very least, a plausible idea. These stormy encounters with friends and relatives have helped many abused women develop into forceful, though illogical, debaters. One of the most amusing quotes I ever encountered was from a young social worker who was leading assertiveness training groups for women. He quit after two years, in complete exasperation, saying that he was burned out from hundreds upon hundreds of hours spent arguing with his "underassertive" clients. His nonbattered women patients were as stubbornly attached to their coping strategies as are victims of domestic abuse.

The battered woman comes from a world where argumentation, irrationality, and defensiveness are a way of life. She is no stranger to verbal and physical conflict, and so she brings a conflictual style into the consulting room. The following annotated exchange between a therapist and an abused woman illustrates the resistances and defenses that are typically encountered in a normal therapy session. Many of the characteristics of individuals with personality disorders that were described in chapter 3 can be seen in this clinical vignette. Note the patient's use of both the moral defense and the splitting defense, her powerful attachment to a bad object, her avoidances, lack of attachment to her children, and her hypersensitivity to criticism.

PT (victoriously): Well, I went to visit Tim this weekend, and he was a perfect gentleman! I told you he was a good person. He just has a temper when he drinks too much. (The patient is in her hopeful self, and her physically abusive boyfriend is seen as an exciting object. All memories of prior abuse are split off.)

TH: I though you told me that you were having trouble getting a baby sitter and that you had to miss your night class two weeks in a row. How could you manage to spend the weekend with Tim? (The patient's urgent dependency needs have a higher priority than her long-term goal of getting an associate degree at a local college.)

PT: Oh, I asked my mother to take the girls. She promised me that she would take good care of them. (The patient's extreme dependency needs cause her to use the splitting defense for a second time. She sees her mother as a good object despite the reality that she was physically abused by her during childhood. These memories are split off in her abused self.)

TH: I hope she doesn't do the same thing to them that she did to you. (Therapist is trying to counter the patient's use of the splitting defense by calling attention to material that had previously emerged in therapy.)

PT: She would never do that stuff to them. If she did I would kill her. (Patient fantasizes an impulsive and aggressive solution to a problem that she created. The needs of her children are less important to her than her own pressing unmet needs.)

TH: How would you know if your mother abused them?

PT: My girls would tell me!

TH: Don't you remember that when you were a little girl you were afraid to tell anyone about your mother? She convinced you that you deserved to be beaten. (This patient had been often beaten as a child with a length of rubber garden hose for minor infractions, and her face was repeatedly scratched by her mother. The therapist is trying to counter patient's use of splitting and focus on the physical danger faced by her children.)

PT: My girls are a lot smarter than I ever was. And you have to face it, I was a wild kid and I got away with a lot of stuff my mother never

knew about. (Patient is trying to defend her actions with a rationalization, and also employs the moral defense to justify her mother's abuse of her.)

TH: Oh? Tell me what you did to deserve having your face scratched
by your mother? I remember you told me that you had to hide out
in the park all day because you were to ashamed to have your
teachers see your face. And when you came home your mother
beat you with the hose for skipping school. (The therapist is trying
to counter the patient's splitting defense, and her use of the moral
defense.)

PT: There you go again! Every thing I do is wrong or stupid! I give up!
Let Allan (the father of her daughters) have the girls! All I want to
do is go and live with Tim. (The patient's low frustration tolerance
and sensitivity to criticism overwhelm her, and she offers an
impulsive and self-destructive solution.)

TH: The last time you told me about Tim he had a restraining order
placed on him for threatening to beat you up. Now you want to go
and live with him. (The therapist keeps working the splitting
defense.)

PT (angrily): I told you he was a perfect gentleman this weekend.
(Patient continues to feel that the therapist is criticizing her by
reminding her of the split off reality that she cannot see.)

This typical exchange illustrates why working with the abused
patient is so challenging. This defensive, argumentative, irresponsible, and avoidant patient was still transfixed by the allure of the
exciting object. Her goal was to meet her own pressing dependency
needs regardless of the consequences to her children. Despite this
patient's history of physical abuse at the hands of her mother, her
urgent needs and powerful defenses allowed her to leave her daughters with their grandmother while she spent time with her boyfriend. Her daughters were not only exposed to danger, but were
repeatedly abandoned when she hastily placed them with various
relatives or friends while she frenetically pursued one futile romantic relationship after another. This dialogue also illustrates the eva-
sive style by which many abused women try to defend themselves
from implied criticism about their actions.

    This particular case had an almost predictable outcome. One of
her daughters was physically abused by the patient's mother. This
daughter showed her bruises to a friend at school, who then told a
teacher. When my patient was informed of this by the school she

was overcome by self-hate and humiliation because she felt that she was exposed as a "bad mother." This is the most dreaded accusation in the borderline mother's vocabulary. The self-hate that was previously split off in her abused self emerged in full force, and was so intense that it prompted her to attempt to take her own life.

This clinical example also illustrates the power of the splitting defense when it is allied to the the individual's unmet needs. This defense does not allow integration of the opposing views of the object that are split apart in the two separate part-selves. My patient's emptiness and overwhelming need for an object was disconnected from key information about her mother and her latest boyfriend. Under circumstances of less need she would not have had to use the splitting defense and would therefore have seen the danger to herself and her daughters.

The dialogue also illustrates that the splitting defense is extremely tenacious and resistant to interference from the outside. The therapist can attempt to use logic, threats, or confrontations to oppose the blindness of the splitting defense. Nothing he says or does will have any effect until the pressure from the patient's dependency needs are reduced. This patient was typical in that my best efforts failed to have an impact, and her splitting defense remained intact. Two months later this same patient planned to leave her older daughter with her mother once again. While this may appear to be malice or stupidity to the observer, it is not. Rather, it is the result of the action of an extremely primitive and powerful defense mechanism. Had that daughter been physically abused by her grandmother, this patient would have been overwhelmed by self-hatred once again. Finally, this example also shows that the abused woman cannot be characterized only by the fact that she is a victim of battering. Rather, her entire personality structure is involved in an endless stream of impulsive need-driven decisions that are based on the malformation of her ego structure due to a deprived childhood.

The Power of Introjection

There are, as I have just outlined, many roadblocks to the patient's successful introjection of positive memories of the supportive therapist. However, when (and if) the process begins, the positive introjects from the therapeutic relationship provide an enormous amount of structure for the inner world of the victim of battering. The new introjects reduce the pressure from the patient's rapacious dependency needs. Once these dependency needs are reduced the patient will have an easier time differentiating from her abuser, and will no longer need to use the splitting defense to hide from the negative aspects of her bad object.

The struggle between the newly internalized memories and the enormous pressures from inner emptiness turns out to be a David and Goliath battle, as it seems impossible for the fifty-minute hour to compensate for a lifetime of neglect. However, each therapy session has a much greater impact than an average interpersonal encounter. I often say to my patients after five or six sessions that I know them better than do either of their parents. In fact, the focused attention, concern, and acceptance of the patient's real self that occurs in six hours of therapy often provides *more* attention, concern, and acceptance than the patient had experienced during all her years of childhood. Many patients tell me that their parents do not have the faintest interest in who they really are. One highly successful professional woman, who had a national reputation in her field, noted that her enormously self-centered father did not know what she did for a living and had never learned to spell her married name!

Over a long series of well-run therapy sessions many patients begin to internalize the feeling that they are being helped by their therapist's efforts. They also begin to imitate the therapist's approach to the problems they present in the therapy hour. The imitation of the therapist occurs both consciously and outside of the patient's awareness. One way to look at the process is to view the patient's problems as a puzzle that she presents to the therapist, who then solves it using his better organized ego. The therapist then offers the solution back to the patient who then reinternalizes it. Over time the patient learns to use the same tactics and approach to problems as does the therapist. Searles (1965) sees this interaction of projection and introjection as central in his work with severely disturbed schizophrenic patients:

> I refer her to the seming circumstance that the therapist, at the deepest levels of the therapeutic interaction, temporarily introjects the patient's pathogenic conflicts and deals with them at an intrapsychic, unconscious as well as a conscious, level, bringing to

bear upon them the capacities of his own relatively strong ego, and then, similarly by introjection, the patient benefits from this intrapsychic therapeutic work which has been accomplished in the therapist. (Searles 1965:214)

The battered woman is not nearly as disturbed, nor as ego deficient, as is the schizophrenic patient. However the process of redeveloping her ego structure follows similar principles. This entire process may sound a bit mysterious, but it is simply a matter of the therapist acting as an auxiliary ego to the patient. The therapist takes on the patient's problems and solves them with his ego, then offers this solution back to the patient. For instance, one of the solutions that the therapist may offer the victim of abuse is that she may be able to tolerate relating to nonabusive men. As I have pointed out, nonabusive men are not interesting to many battered women because they do not emit the alternation of exciting and rejecting behaviors that stimulate her two part-selves. However, as time passes the therapist may be able to imagine a way for the abused woman to become interested in less exciting (and more demanding) men. The therapist's ability to imagine the possibility, along with the internalizations of the therapist as a nonexciting, yet gratifying, object allows this new behavior to become a possibility in the future. The gradual introjection of the therapist's view, along with positive memories from the ongoing therapeutic relationship, helps to support her identity while she begins to relate to this new, mysterious, and frightening group of men.

Over time the therapist's efforts to help the patient creates an assurance in her that she will be related to with interest, respect, and concern. This expectation in her begins to build a collection of holding-soothing introjects. These memories, along with the specific techniques introjected from the therapist's "loaned" ego, constitute the process of "reparenting." It is a strange concept to use when the patient is forty years old, but it can occur in patients of any age, because their internal world is still empty and in need of introjects.

Introjection and the Process of Identity Building

The battering victim often does not know who she really is. Her original objects may have misidentified her so completely that her organic talents, interests, and proclivities were completely ignored and thus never flowered. In many instances the child is identified as being identical to someone with whom she has no real resemblance. Often parents will project their own inner world onto the child, who might, for instance, be identified as being just like "Aunt Martha" or some other relative with whom she has no organic commonalty. In very primitive families all "badness" is projected onto one child who then "contains" all the sins of the family.

An important aspect of the therapist's task when helping the victim of abuse to build a firm identity is for him to formulate a vision of the patient that is congruent with her talents and interests. That is, the therapist has to guide the development of the patient's sense of self by accurately mirroring back what he sees. Each patient presents enough "self" in the therapeutic encounter for the therapist to develop an accurate vision of her potential. Loewald (1960) sees this aspect of the therapist's task as part of the reparenting process:

> The parent-child relationship can serve as a model here. The parent ideally is in an empathic relationship of understanding the child's particular stage of development, yet ahead in his vision of the child's future and mediating this vision to the child in dealing with him. This vision, informed by the parent's own experience and knowledge of growth and future, is, ideally, a more articulate and more integrated version of the core of being which the child presents to the parent. (Loewald 1960:20)

The therapist has to gradually present this vision to the battered woman, and allow enough time for her ego to internalize this view of herself as she develops. This is a relatively active process, one in which the therapist, again, carries a considerable burden.

Fostering Differentiation of the Abused Woman from Her Exciting/Rejecting Objects

Now that the problems and possibilities surrounding the process of introjection have been discussed, it is time to focus on the second therapeutic task, differentiating the patient from her abusive partner. This is the second major goal of the therapist who works with the abused woman. The previous dialogue between patient and therapist illustrated the problems inherent in this task. The therapeutic goal of separating the battered woman from her abusive partner will be resisted by the patient, since even minor periods of separation are experienced as abandonments. Her fundamental inability to operate as an independent human being is the psychological disability that keeps her trapped in a relationship with her abusive partner. There is no amount of force the therapist can exert on the patient that will motivate her to leave her abuser. It is analogous to trying to force a neglected child to leave his family. Once again the therapist must rely on his only tool: the gradual internalization of positive introjects that accumulate over time in the patient's interior world. The therapist has to refrain from putting too much pressure on the abused patient until she has some inner strength. She simply cannot let her abuser go until such time as she has internalized enough of the therapist's support to keep her sense of self intact as she individuates.

The Patient's Resistance to the Process of Differentiation

At the outset of therapy even the most innocent and circumspect examination of the patient's history will be screened for any implication that she should leave her partner. It must be remembered that these patients are petrified by the fear that they may be forced to leave their life-giving object. If the therapist takes the simplistic tactic that the patient should leave her abusive partner immediately, "for her own good," then the therapist is advertising the fact that she doesn't have a basic understanding of the dynamics of the battered woman, and will be unable to offer her much help. The undertrained but well-meaning therapist will be just another annoyance to the battered woman, who is already overwhelmed by people telling her what to do.

The skilled therapist understands that she must work with the inner dynamics of the abused woman. Chapter 4 illustrated that the internal structure of the abused woman is a complex and fluid system. It is technically difficult to intervene with change-producing strategies when the therapist is aware of the patient's complex inner structure, and nearly impossible when she is not. Many unsophisticated therapists fail in their efforts to help abused women because of their lack of knowledge of the typical split ego structure that dominates the inner worlds of these patients.

Each statement the therapist makes adds to the strength of one, or the other, internal part-selves (the hopeful self or the abused self) of the abused woman. Poorly thought out statements can tip the precarious internal balance between the two part-selves, and may provoke the patient to call on the splitting defense. Let me illustrate this danger by returning to the example of Jennifer. My lengthy, detailed, and supportive examination of the many childhood incidents of abuse that she suffered seemed to be an appropriate therapeutic approach. However, as my examination of her history went on, Jennifer's abused self became stronger and stronger, because of my overt validation of her past experiences. My support tipped the internal balance between the two part-selves because it made her abused self stronger relative to her hopeful self. The newly powerful abused self was then able to hold onto a vision of her mother as a truly abusive and hateful person, and this perception produced an abandonment panic in Jennifer. Her despair forced her to use the splitting defense to repress her abused self and to simultaneously reinstate her hopeful self in the dominant position. This unrealistic part-self allowed her to return home to her mother, thus temporarily relieving her sense of abandonment. My negative characterization of her mother thwarted progress, provoked an unnecessary episode of acting out, and ultimately convinced Jennifer that I was more trouble than I was worth.

The shift in the strength of the two part-selves is not a problem in a normal person. The normal individual does not have to contend with two competing and opposite part-selves. Indeed, the normal person feels that the world contains many alternative sources of love and support because her early experience of the world was filled with love. In contrast, the battered woman does not believe that there are any alternatives to her abusive partner. She is intensely focused on her one-and-only life-giving object. This brings us back to Fairbairn's first principle—that the abused and neglected child needs the parent *more* than does the well-loved and emotionally supported child. This fundamental truth points out one of the most "unfair" aspects of defective parenting in terms of helping the victim of severe abuse later on in life. Those battered women who experienced the most severe developmental deprivation are the patients who are most desperately attached to their abusive partners and who are least accepting of help that is aimed at making them more independent.

A Therapeutic Approach Designed to Aid the Victim's Differentiation from Her Abuser

The previous discussion of introjection of memories from the therapeutic relationship emphasized the key role of that process in the rehabilitation of the victim of abuse. In reality there is little concrete action the therapist can take to foster differentiation, as separation from the abuser is dependent upon the state of the patient's inner resources (introjects) and upon the strength of her splitting defense. The therapist's most important job is avoid making the fundamental error of forcing the patient to differentiate too early, since this misguided effort will cause either a regression or termination of the therapeutic relationship.

The therapist's introduction to the patient is most likely provoked by difficulties with her abusive partner, since battered women seldom enter therapy when they are not threatened with abandonment. As I mentioned in the previous section, the therapist's first job is to form an alliance with the patient. The abused self is the part-self that is dominant when there are difficulties with the abusing object, and this is the part-self that the therapist initially encounters. I have *never* been contacted by an abused woman when she was dominated by her hopeful self, for when she experiences the world from that part-self she is cut off from memories of her pain.

Initially the therapist simply relates to the patient's abusive self, and gathers information about her life without overemphasizing the "badness" of her object. The therapist must keep in mind that the "reality" that is developed between himself and the patient's abused self is an entirely different "reality" as compared to the relationship that will emerge with the patient's hopeful self. The therapist cannot believe in either reality, because both of the part-selves have an unrealistic view of the abuser. This topic will be discussed further in the following section on integration.

The second step, after the therapist has developed an alliance with the abused self, is to gently confront the patient's use of the moral defense. This is less important (and less difficult) than confronting the patient's use of the splitting defense. The therapist's examination of the patient's use of the moral defense helps the process of differentiation by contrasting the position taken by the patient and her abusive partner with the therapist's perspective regarding the "reasonableness" of the abuse directed toward her. To begin the process the therapist must solicit a problem from the patient's childhood in which she blamed herself for her parents abuse of her. It is best to begin with a distant event as this does not pressure the abused woman to see that she is using the very same defense to hide from the "badness" of her current partner. The therapist simply reviews family events in which the patient was blamed or blamed herself for the failures of her parents. Then the therapist has to reexamine the situation and contrast the family acceptance of the view that the patient was somehow responsible for events that were, in reality, far beyond her control, with her more realistic view. The next step is to explain to the patient that her use of the moral defense was the way that she justified her continued attachment to her abusive/neglectful parents. The final, and critical, step is to apply the same schema to the current battering event that has just occurred between the partners. The therapist contrasts the abuser's position, which is supported by the patient's use of the moral defense, with the reality that no adult "deserves" to be beaten for anything. Once again the therapist must not press too strongly, because if the abused woman assumes that she is supposed to leave her abuser simply because she is *being told* that she is using the same defense that she used in childhood, it will cause her to flee therapy. The therapist has to allow enough time for the abused woman to understand the concept fully and be able to apply it consistently to past and present situations in her life.

Where is the abused woman in this process? At the outset she does not know what position is real, and she will vacillate between the two opposing positions like a child caught between warring parents. She might go back to her abuser with the therapist's explanation of the moral defense and ask him if it is true. This is often the state of the battered woman's ego when she first begins therapy. I have noted, again and again, that these patients "can't tell their friends from their enemies."

Another major impediment to the patient's separation from her abuser is her irrational but powerful sense of guilt for abandoning her partner. At some level the abused woman recognizes that her partner is an infant clothed in an adult body. A similar observation has been made by Walker:

> Battered women sense their men's desperation, loneliness, and alienation from the rest of society. They see themselves as the bridge to their men's emotional well-being. Nearly half of the women interviewed reported that their husband's sanity deteriorated after they left them. (Walker 1979:68)

This issue was mentioned in chapter 5. Many battered women had similar experiences and perceptions of their original parents. At some level they recognized that their parents were emotionally handicapped, and this awareness, and the guilt attached to it, acted as another impediment to separation from the family. The abused woman feels responsible for the well-being of her violent partner, and assumes that he will either deteriorate or perish if she leaves him. Naturally, this powerful guilt complicates the process of separation enormously, and the therapist must challenge the patient's sense of responsibility for the well-being of the man who is beating her.

The therapist must also strengthen the victim of abuse in terms of her normal daily interpersonal functioning with her partner. The victim of abuse is not only used to being hurt physically but interpersonally as well. The battered woman is not able to defend herself verbally from accusations made by her partner, and this inability to stand up for her rights promotes both the fear and the respect that she typically has for the rejecting objects in her life. The patient is accustomed to losing all her interpersonal arguments with her partner because she assumes she is the source of all badness (the moral defense), and because her use of the splitting defense does not allow her to hold to a single position during these exchanges. Her unstable perceptions, and her inability to dismiss her partner's alternative view, results in a loss of confidence in her shifting perceptions of reality. In some respects she is like a prizefighter who has to go into the ring with one arm tied behind his back. The effects of these two powerful defenses leave the battered woman in an interpersonally defenseless position. Finally, she also fears that if she should happen to "win" her long-term fight with her abuser she risks losing him for good.

The therapist's task is to strengthen the patient's interpersonal functioning by teaching her tactics that will make her more effective in dealing with the people in her world. Again, this has to be a gradual process, because of the patient's fear of the loss of her partner. She has to acquire positive introjects that support her sense of self before she will be willing to defeat her abusive partner. Let me illustrate this "skills training" process with a former patient. In this case the patient was a fifty-year-old woman who had suffered innumerable physical assaults during her first marriage. Despite her escape from that marriage she continued to have difficulty dealing with her extremely abusive and rejecting mother who used to punish her during childhood by locking her in an unheated outbuilding on their farm. Her father had died and left her an extensive collection of valuable antiques. Her mother refused to allow her to take the antiques to her own home because she claimed her daughter would not care for them properly. My patient asked her mother for them again and again, only to be refused. The patient's mother also demanded that her daughter pick her up at her home for weekly visits that consisted of nonstop criticism of my patient. Naturally she dreaded these visits, but her massive dependency needs did not allow her to protect herself from her mother's aggression. She would think of things to say during her mother's abusive onslaughts, but was unable to verbalize them. She feared that her mother would attack her for being a bad, selfish, or irresponsible daughter. I used role-playing with this patient, took her role, and voiced her unverbalized feeling toward her mother—expressing feelings she feared would cause her to be abandoned once and for all. I would then ask her to play her mother's role and retaliate against me as much as possible:

TH (playing role of patient):   Well, Mom, I see that you are wielding your power over me by not giving up the antiques that Father wanted me to have. This is nothing new. You have pulled the same trick on me my whole life. I used to think that if I gave in to your needs that someday you would come forth with all the love and support that I desperately longed for. I now see that I can't lose something that doesn't exist! You fooled me into believing that you were a loving mother, and I helped you by fooling myself. I used to believe that you were filled with love and had wisely withheld it from me because I was not important or successful enough.

PT (playing the role of her mother): You little witch. Would you tell me once and for all why you are such are a terrible daughter? You don't visit me enough, and all the horrible lies you just told about me prove what a horrible person you are. I was a perfect mother.

TH (playing daughter): You were the perfect mother! You locked me in the shed time after time perfectly. You called me names perfectly. You pulled my hair perfectly.

This type of repeated role-playing demonstrates to the patient that it is possible to tell the truth and not give in to the pressure from the rejecting parent or partner. It validates the reality that the patient's innermost beliefs about the bad object are correct. In this particular case my patient was able to defend herself from her mother's frequent accusations after six or seven sessions. She was no longer fearful of the abandonment that her mother had previously used as a threat when she fought against her mother's criticisms. Abandonment became less terrifying for this patient when she realized that she had already been abandoned, and when she felt she could depend on her therapist. Interestingly, this patient (as well as many others) told me that she "knew" the truth about her mother all along but could not face the massive feelings of abandonment that would follow the acceptance of these truths.

During our work this patient shifted her dependency needs away from her mother and onto me. Within a short time she lost interest in phoning her mother, and she no longer carried out her weekly visits. Within two weeks of this shift my patient was surprised by the arrival of a van containing all the antiques that were left to her by her father. This is absolutely typical of the abusive parent. They are extremely sensitive to their power over their child, and will change their tactics in order to regain the power they once enjoyed the moment the child begins to slip away. It is not possible to say with certainty whether this shift was a consequence of the "training" or of the shift of the patient's dependency needs away from the bad object. However, my experience strongly suggests that "skills training" is of no value until the patient has enough positive introjects to face the sure abandonment that will follow if they employ a firmer position in relationship to their bad object. Once again, this example illustrates the reality that there is an intimate tie between ill-treatment in childhood and abuse in adulthood.

Integration of the Patient's Ego Structure

The third therapeutic goal when working with the victim of abuse is to diminish the patient's use of the splitting defense, which protects her from the harsh reality of her abusive partner. The actual task of the therapist is to mend the two separate part-object images of the abuser into a single, stable image. A second goal, usually accomplished at the same time, is for the therapist to facilitate the process of mending the patient's two part-selves (hopeful and abused) into a single sense of self. The therapist who works with this population has to have an excellent model of the patient's inner world, for he will have to deal with many areas of the patient's ego simultaneously.

The patient's use of the splitting defense causes endless mischief in her life. It must be kept in mind that the purpose of the splitting defense is to keep the victim of battering unaware of the huge collection of painful memories that interfere with her attachment to her abuser. The splitting defense allows her to hide from the hate and hopelessness of the relationship. The process of introjection of positive memories of the therapist has to be well underway before the patient will be able to tolerate any confrontation of her use of the splitting defense. Again, introjection is the key to the repair of the abused woman's damaged ego. Neither differentiation nor integration can proceed until some number of supportive memories have been internalized.

The Patient's Attempt to Split the Therapist The very reliability and availability of the therapist works to undermine the patient's splitting defense. Simply stated, the patient begins to expect that her therapist will be available to her every week for their therapy session. Even a minimally skilled and alert therapist is able to offer more support to the patient than did her original objects or her abusive partner. There appears to be absolutely no reason for the abused woman to split the therapist into "gratifying" and "rejecting" parts since he/she is available, consistent, and supportive. There is no apparent "badness" in the therapeutic relationship from which the patient needs to hide. Despite this, the severely deprived patient *will split* the therapist into good and bad parts. This is particularly true at the outset of therapy, when the patient is still extremely needy and sensitive. Anything the therapist says that doesn't *exactly* agree with the patient will be split off into the "bad part-therapist." It is not uncommon for the abused patient to interrupt the therapist constantly and "correct" his statements because the patient cannot tolerate any reality that reduces her perilously low self-esteem or that threatens her relationship with her abuser. This was illustrated in the previous dialogue in which the patient corrected the therapist's view of her abusive boyfriend. At that moment the patient was experiencing the therapist as a rejecting object.

When the patient splits the therapist into "good" and "bad" parts she is free to attack the "bad" part-therapist with a vengeance. Again, this is due to the perception that there are two separate therapists. This is yet another reason why the abused woman is a challenging patient. It is particularly galling for the naive and well-meaning therapist to be attacked by the enraged patient when the therapist makes *what the patient has defined as a "mistake."* The patient feels completely justified about her aggressive behavior, just as her abusive partner felt justified when he physically attacked her. The battered woman's sudden shift of position from dependent-gratitude to aggressive-rejection is identical to other borderline patients who Kernberg (1980) described as behaving "ruthlessly" in the transference.

The therapist's job is to counter the patient's tendency to split him into separate "good" and "bad" parts. If the patient becomes excessively angry toward the therapist she should calmly point out how quickly the patient has forgotten all of her past efforts, and how willing the patient is to discard the therapist. The patient who uses the splitting defense will turn against the therapist the moment he feels the pressure from unmet needs. In some cases it is also advisable to explain the process of splitting, however, intellectual understanding of the defense probably does little to help integration.

Integration of the Patient's View of Herself, and of Her Abuser

A more potent source of potential benefit to the patient's split view of her abusing object is the therapist's consistent and integrated view of the abuser. This view of the abuser will be at odds with the unrealistic views contained in both the patient's hopeful and abused selves. The therapist will disagree with the patient's fantasy in her hopeful self, which imagines that the abuser contains the potential to love her in the future. The continuous tension between the therapist's view and the patient's hopeful-self view of the abuser as an exciting object will help the patient "remember" parts of him she would prefer to ignore. That is, the therapist's view will begin to challenge the patient's hopeful-self view, and this process of comparing the two views helps to integrate the exciting part-object and the rejecting part-object into a single "whole-object" view of the partner.

Interestingly, the therapist's view of the abuser will also be at variance with the patient's vision of him when she is dominated by her abused self. When the abused self is dominant her partner will appear to be an enormously potent, demonlike entity, one who has vast powers and cannot be opposed. As I have mentioned, the abused woman takes the rejecting object very seriously, and he is both feared and respected. In contrast, the therapist's view of the abuser is that he is a weak and emotionally infantile man who has learned to enslave the patient by alternating from hopeful to rejecting behaviors. He has no power in the world at large, yet he has almost unlimited power over his victim.

Another source of integration is the therapist's consistent view of the patient, which affects the patient's split sense of self rather than her split view of the abuser. The therapist's consistent view of the patient gives her a single view of herself to internalize, one that is often at odds with the temporary view of herself that she brings into the consulting room. This is a different process from the previously described presentation of a "vision" to the patient who has a weak identity. This is a more straightforward process in which the therapist simply holds onto a single view of the patient, and contrasts her view with the patient's fluid and chaotic sense of self. The abused patient typically presents herself as a number of separate people. One is the injured, abandoned, victimized self that resides in the abused self. Another is the guilty and deserving-of-abuse self that emerges from the patient's use of the moral defense. Other selves include the simplistic revenge-driven fanatic self who wants to kill all abusers and sees the world in black and white terms. All these selves emerge at one time or another in the therapy of the abused woman. The therapist has to remind the patient of her "other selves," which have been present at other times in the consulting room. The therapist must make each split off separate self more a part of the patient's "central ego," which Fairbairn defined as the realistic self that is well integrated and unchanging.

The Timing and Ultimate Outcome
of Therapeutic Interventions

Now that the three basic ego processes have been discussed, it is useful to examine the timing of the therapist's interventions. The therapist's model of the human personality will determine when and
how she intervenes. There are moments when opportunities are present, and others when conditions make intervention futile and self-
defeating. Some models are better than others at understanding the
underlying processes of the battering scenario, and the better models give the therapist a more detailed plan for the intervention
process. The reward for the mental health professional who uses a
superior model is that she will be more effective in impacting the
patient than colleagues who use less accurate models.

There is a very small window during the third stage of the battering scenario that allows for intervention if the therapist works with
both members of the couple. That moment occurs when the abuser
has split back to his hopeful self, and when the victim is still in her
abused self. The therapist can use access to the victim as tool to
force compliance from the temporarily contrite abuser. This is not
the method that I use personally, however, the model does accurately predict that this is the moment when the therapist has maximum influence.

Later interventions during the third stage of the battering cycle
will be futile and self-defeating if they come after the victim has
forcefully split back into her hopeful self. Once the victim's perceptions are dominated by this part-self, she can no longer see any "badness" in the man who just beat her. She is excited about the possibility of love in her partner, and anyone who attempts to disturb this
fantasy will be rejected. This model also predicts that the therapist's
influence (which is derived from his gradual introjection into the
inner world of the patient) will be low at the outset of the relationship. Without a relatively long-term relationship with the patient,
the therapist approaches her without any interpersonal leverage.
Walker (1979) has observed the difficulty of intervention during the
latter part of the the third stage. The following quote also illustrates
how her choice of language attempts to minimize the battered
woman's pathology by claiming that the rewards of marriage (an
entirely commendable source of motivation) are the source of the

blind drive to return to the abuser. In fact the motivation is far more primitive—akin to the abandoned infant's frenetic drive to be reunited with her mother:

> Since most of the rewards of being married or coupled occur during phase three for the battered woman, this is the time when it is most difficult for her to make a decision to end the relationship. Unfortunately, it is also the time during which helpers usually see her. When she resists leaving the relationship and pleads that she really loves him, she bases her reference to the current loving phase-three behavior rather than on the more painful phase-one or phase-two behavior. . . . The women interviewed consistently admitted, although somewhat shamefacedly, that they loved their men dearly during this phase. The effect of their men's generosity, dependability, helpfulness, and genuine interest cannot be minimized. (Walker 1979:69)

Thus the latter part of the third phase of the battering cycle (after the victim has split back into the hopeful self) is one of the least opportune moments for the therapist to intervene in the battering scenario. It is impossible for the therapist to aid, cajole, or force the victim of abuse to integrate her split view of her abuser at this moment. If the therapist is required to intervene at this stage in the cycle, the model that I have outlined would recommend that he *avoid* direct discussion of the abuser and begin simply to penetrate the victim's blunted awareness that there are others in the universe to whom she can safely relate. If the well-meaning human services worker overemphasizes how vicious and cruel the batterer was during the prior two phases, the victim will be deeply offended, because those memories are no longer available to her. In addition to dissipating what little effectiveness he might have had, the therapist's attempt to challenge the victim's view of the abuser might cause the patient to reject all future contact.

When the therapeutic process does go well, it is possible to restructure the ego of many battered women in three to five years of individual therapy. This assumes that the therapist has a good working model that helps him withstand the pressure from the frequent reversals and from patient aggression that is directed toward the therapist during the treatment process. It also assumes that the patient has the insurance or financial resources to pay for the long course of treatment. If she sees a therapist in a public mental health center, that therapist must be willing to stick out the years of treatment and not become overwhelmed by the dozens of other similar patients he has. In either case, the odds are against full repair of the disorder, even if the four factors that impede introjection are swept aside by the therapist's training and skill. It is a venture that has many obstacles in its way because of the sheer amount of time it takes to repair characterological disorders. Long-term treatment of the abused woman demands that the patient think of the future rather than the present and lead a stable life that allows her to stay in one geographical area for many years. She also needs the discipline to bear up under what seems like criticism from her therapist. All of these characteristics are in short supply in both the external and the internal world of the battered woman.

A Model for the Future

It is clear from my discussion of the difficulties in the treatment of battered women that individual treatment of each and every victim will not begin to address this problem, which has now reached crisis proportions. As I have noted, the treatment of each victim is enormously time-consuming, expensive, and does not insure success. It is somewhat paradoxical that I have developed a treatment program for severe character disorders that include battered women only to conclude that it is an enterprise ultimately doomed to failure. My opinion is based on the bedrock reality that the vast majority of abused women will never get a fraction of the specialized help that they require to restructure their damaged sense of self. The notion that we can solve a problem like battering by "repairing" each individual who is afflicted by abuse without rectifying the underlying social problems, ignores everything we know about the conquest of similar human dilemmas. It is a futile enterprise, because treating each individual does nothing to prevent the simultaneous development of hundreds more cases. Large-scale social change has to occur so that society no longer "manufactures" thousand upon thousands of abusers and victims every year:

> Further, as the history of public health methods (that emphasize social change) has clearly established, no mass disease or disorder afflicting humankind has ever been eliminated by attempts at

treating afflicted individuals. Changing the incidence of emotional disorders will require large-scale political and social changes affecting the rates of injustice, powerlessness, and exploitation, none of which is affected by individual psychotherapy.

(Albee 1990:370)

A second intractable reality that eliminates individual psychotherapy as an effective answer to the epidemic of battering is the fact that there are not enough mental health professionals to deal with the victims of abuse, and the gap between numbers of abused women and mental health professionals is getting worse rather than better.

> How many therapists actually are available for the vast sea of troubled people? Kiesler and Sulkin (1987) have calculated the total number of (full-time equivalent) therapists to be about 45,000. This may be a conservative estimate, but even if we add to this figure the unlicensed and unregulated personal counselors, yoga instructors, teachers of meditation, pastoral counselors, and school guidance personnel we have only doubled or tripled the total number. . . . But we must remind ourselves that even if there were twenty times as many psychotherapists there would be no reduction in the incidence of problems, a majority of which are caused by poverty, powerlessness, exploitation and social injustice. (Albee 1990:373)

I have already alluded to another problem, inherent in the attempt to repair every afflicted individual, which is the preparation, knowledge, and skill of those mental health professionals who deal with the victims of battering. The very nature of the disorder, its severity and resistance to treatment decreases the chances of success, even if the abused woman does find a willing mental health professional to work with her. In my experience, I have found that very few clinicians *know* about the dynamics of the battered woman, and many of these individuals specifically avoid this population because they are so difficult to deal with therapeutically. Those battered women that do find a therapist are usually dealt with by well-meaning mental health professionals who are often not equipped to to bear up under the frustration, the complexities, and the reversals of direction that are part of nearly every course of treatment. I have been told by many colleagues who deal with severe character disorders that they are "burnt-out" after five to ten years in the field. These practitioners are exposed to intolerable levels of frustration of their efforts both because the models they use do not prescribe interventions that lead to success and because character problems are enormously difficult to deal with under the best of conditions.

The problem, as I see it, is our culture's almost unbelievable blindness to the long-term effects of abusive or neglectful childhoods. We, as a society, treasure stories about those few examples of success that are won against all odds, and willfully refuse to see that for every abused and neglected child who "makes" it there are thousands who do not. I do not want this book to give the reader the same type of false hope. The goal of this book is to educate professionals and interested laypersons about the dynamics of the abuse scenario. The model that I have described is far superior to the existing model of the disorder that is currently used. It clearly explains the previously misunderstood dynamics of both individuals involved in any given battering scenario. However, a better model *of treatment* is not going to solve the problem of domestic abuse. In fact, the complexities involved in the treatment of the battered woman that have been described make things appear more difficult than before. The real value of this model, as compared to the model presented by Walker, is that it focuses on the absolute importance of the child's early experiences in life. That is, it offers a rationale and a focus on the possibility of prevention of the disorder. We can now reliably demonstrate that certain types of early childhood deprivations guarantee that the exposed child will seek out in his or her adulthood partners who recreate the original style of emotional deprivation. This knowledge should guide us toward new social policies that minimize the possibility that future generations of children will be exposed to the conditions that would shape them into future abusers or victims of abuse.

I do not want this "new and improved" model of the dynamics of domestic violence to be used as another false hope for the "cure" of this social epidemic. It may impact a few victims of abuse, however, the overwhelming majority of battered women will never find a therapist, let alone one who has heard of this book. The fact that a few mental health professionals do know how to treat victims of abuse will not in any way stem the tide of women who are beaten every year. The real issue is not the existence of a better form of therapy but rather a model that points to specific areas of child development that must be improved if we are to solve this human dilemma. If our society begins to focus on prevention of the specific types of family problems that we now know lead to the endless continuation of abuse from generation to generation then we will have a chance of impacting this enormous problem. However, given the state of our current social policies, and the emphasis on parental rights that effectively block all substantial intervention into dysfunctional families until the children are nearly destroyed, we as a society are assured of an endless supply of children who will be subjected to developmentally damaging experiences that guarantee they will emerge as either the next crop of abusers or as victims of abuse.

REFERENCES

Adler, G. 1985. *Borderline Psychopathology and Its Treatment.* New York: Jason Aronson.

Ainsworth, M. D. 1977. "Social Development in the First Year of Life: Maternal Influences on Infant-Mother Attachment." In J. M. Tanner, ed., *Developments in Psychiatric Research.* London: Tavistock.

Albee, G. W. 1990. "The Futility of Psychotherapy." *Journal of Mind and Behavior* 11:369–384.

Armstrong-Perlman, E. 1991. "The Allure of the Bad Object." *Free Association* 2:343–356.

Barnett, O. W. and A. D. LaViolette. 1993. *It Could Happen To Anyone.* Newbury Park, Cal.: Sage.

Beck, M. and G. Carroll. 1979. "The Strange Case of Annie Perry." *Newsweek,* p. 37. December 31.

Bowlby, J. 1988. *A Secure Base.* New York: Basic.

Breuer, J. and S. Freud. 1895. *Studies On Hysteria.* Vol. 2. The Standard Edition of the Complete Psychological Works of Sigmund Freud. Ed. James Strachey. London: Hogarth Press.

Browne, A. 1992. "Violence Against Women, Relevance for Medical Practitioners." *Journal of the American Medical Association* 267:3,184–3,189.

Celani, D. P. 1993. *The Treatment of the Borderline Patient: Applying Fairbairn's Object Relations Theory in the Clinical Setting.* Madison, Conn.: International Universities Press.

Cowan, C. and M. Kinder. 1985. *Smart Women Foolish Choices.* New York: Signet.

Drinka, G. F. 1984. *The Birth of Neurosis.* New York: Simon and Schuster.

Erikson, E. H. 1950. *Childhood and Society.* New York: Norton.

Fairbairn, W. R. D. 1940. "Schizoid Factors in the Personality." In W. R. D. Fairbairn, *Psychoanalytic Studies of the Personality,* pp. 3–27. London: Routledge and Kegan Paul, 1952.

— 1941. "A Revised Psychopathology of the Psychoses and Psychoneuroses." *International Journal of Psycho-Analysis* 22:250–279.

— 1943. "The Repression and the Return of Bad Objects (with Special Reference to the `War Neuroses')." *British Journal of Medical Psychology* 19:327–341.

— 1944. "Endopsychic Structure Considered in Terms of Object-Relationships." *International Journal of Psycho-Analysis*, vol. 25, parts 1 and 2.

— 1946. "Object-Relationships and Dynamic Structure." *International Journal of Psycho-Analysis*, vol. 27, parts 1 and 2.

— 1951. "A Synopsis of the Development of the Author's Views Regarding the Structure of the Personality." In W. R. D. Fairbairn, *Psychoanalytic Studies of the Personality*, pp. 162–179. London: Routledge and Kegan Paul, 1952.

— 1963. "Synopsis of an Object-Relations Theory of the Personality." *International Journal of Psycho-Analysis* 44:224–255.

Freud, S. 1920. *Beyond the Pleasure Principle.* 18:7–64. The Standard Edition of the Complete Psychological Works of Sigmund Freud. Ed. James Strachey. London: Hogarth Press.

— 1924. *The Economic Problem of Masochism.* 19:159–170. The Standard Edition of the Complete Psychological Works of Sigmund Freud. Ed. James Strachey. London: Hogarth Press.

Foward, S. and J. Torres. 1986. *Men Who Hate Women and the Women Who Love Them.* New York: Bantam.

George, C. and M. Main. 1979. "Social Interactions of Young Abused Children: Approach, Avoidance, and Aggression." *Child Development* 50:306–318.

Greenson, R. R. 1978. *Explorations in Psychoanalysis.* New York: International Universities Press.

Guntrip, H. 1975. "My Experiences in Analysis with Fairbairn and Winnicott." *International Review of Psychoanalysis* 2:145–156.

Hamilton, N. G. 1988. *Self and Others, Object Relations Theory in Practice.* Northvale, N.J.: Jason Aronson.

Harlow, H. F. 1986. "Love and Aggression." In C. M. Harlow, ed., *From Learning to Love: The Selected Papers of H. F. Harlow.* New York: Prager.

Kernberg, O. 1966. "Structural derivatives of object relations." *International Journal of Psycho-Analysis* 47(2):236–253.

— 1980. *Internal World and External Reality.* New York: Jason Aronson.

Kiesler, C. A. and A. E. Sulkin. 1987. *Mental Hospitalization: Myths and Facts About a National Crisis.* Newbury Park, Cal.: Sage.

Langs, R. J. 1973a. *The Technique of Psychoanalytic Psychotherapy.* Vol. 1. New York: Jason Aronson.

— 1973b. *The Technique of Psychoanalytic Psychotherapy.* Vol. 2. New York: Jason Aronson.

Leo, J. 1981. "A Sad Baffling Dependency," p. 45. *Time*, April 6.

Little, M. I. 1981. *Transference Neurosis and Transference Psychosis.* New York: Jason Aronson.

Loewald, H. 1960. "On the Therapeutic Action of Psychoanalysis." *International Journal of Psycho-Analysis* 41:16–33.

Lomas, P. 1987. *The Limits of Interpretation.* New York: Penguin.

Mahler, M., F. Pine, and A. Bergman. 1975. *The Psychological Birth of the Human Infant.* New York: Basic.

Main, M. and C. George. 1985. "Response of Abused and Disadvantaged Toddlers to Distress in Age-Mates: A Study in the Day Care Setting". *Developmental Psychology* 21:407–412.

Marzuk, P., K. Tardiff, and C. Hirsch. 1992. "The Epidemiology of Murder-Suicide." *Journal of the American Medical Association* 267:3,179–3,183.

Masterson, J. F. 1988. *The Search for the Real Self.* New York: Free Press.

Norwood, R. 1985. *Women Who Love Too Much.* New York: St. Martin's.

Page, H. 1885. *Injuries of the Spine and Spinal Cord and Nervous Shock.* Philadelphia: Blackiston.

Porter, K. A. 1970. *The Collected Essays and Occasional Writings of Katherine Anne Porter.* Boston: Houghton Miffin.

Rayner, E. 1991. *The Independent Mind in British Psychoanalysis.* Northvale, N.J.: Jason Aronson.

Rey, J. H. 1979. "Schizoid Phenomena in the Borderline." In J. Le Boit and A. Capponi, eds., *Advances in Psychotherapy of the Borderline Patient,* pp. 449–484. New York: Jason Aronson.

Roth, P. 1967. *Portnoy's Complaint.* New York: Bantam.

Searles, H. F. 1965. *Collected Papers on Schizophrenia and Related Topics.* New York: International Universities Press.

Seinfeld, J. 1990. *The Bad Object.* Northvale, N.J.: Jason Aronson.

Shengold, L. 1989. *Soul Murder.* New York: Ballantine.

Sugg, N. and T. Inui. 1992. "Primary Care Physicians' Response to Domestic Violence: Opening Pandora's Box." *Journal of the American Medical Association* 267:3,157–3,160.

Walker, L. E. 1979. *The Battered Woman.* New York: Harper and Row.

Watson, J. B. and Rayner, R. 1920. "Conditioned Emotional Reactions." *Journal of Experimental Psychology* 3(1):1–14.

Winnicott, D. 1986. *Home Is Where We Start From.* New York: Norton.

Wolkind, S., Hall, F., and Pawlby, S. 1977. "Individual Differences in Mothering Behavior. In P. J. Graham, ed., *Epidemiological Approaches to Child Psychiatry,* pp. 107–123. New York: Academic Press.

Zahn-Waxler, C., R. A. King, and M. Radke-Yarrow. 1979. "Childrearing and Childrens' Prosocial Initations Toward Victims of Distress." *Child Development* 50:319–330.